VIBRATIONAL
RAINDROP
TECHNIQUE

Third Edition

CHRISTI BONDS-GARRETT
M.A., M.D.

Third Edition
1 3 5 7 9 11 13 15 17 19 20 18 16 14 12 10 8 6 4 2

Life Science Publishing
1.800.336.6308
www.DiscoverLSP.com

By Christi Bonds-Garrett, M.D.
Illustrations by Christi Bonds-Garrett, M.D.
Printed in the United States of America

Disclaimer:
The information contained in this book is for educational purposes only. It is not provided to diagnose, prescribe, or treat any condition of the body. The information in this book should not be used as a substitute for medical counseling with a health professional. Neither the author nor publisher accepts responsibility for such use. In cases where inflammation may be present, exercise extreme caution in the application of essential oils to the skin.

DEDICATED TO GARY YOUNG,

VISIONARY CREATOR OF RAINDROP

TECHNIQUE; AND TO MARY YOUNG,

THE HARMONICS BEHIND THE HEALING

About the Cover Art for Vibrational Raindrop Technique, 3rd Edition:

The other day in my medical acupuncture clinic, I was starting to apply essential oils to a new client's back before using tuning forks along his spine. Out of the blue, he started telling me how he was reminded of the feathering that his ancestors did for healing.

"What do you mean?" I asked. Not many clients mention the word "feathering" when we talk. And Jeffrey did not know anything about Raindrop Technique, in fact had never heard of it.

"My grandmother who raised me was a full-blooded Lakota. She often told me stories about how her People would go north above the Canadian border, to reach the Northern Lights. Those who were ill would lie down on the ground in order to absorb the healing energy which the Northern Lights put into the ground." My goodness, I thought; this is exactly what Dr. Gary Young has written about the origins of Raindrop Technique!

"As the Northern lights came," Jeffrey continued, "the healers would strip you down and lay you on the ground. They believed the energy from the Lights came up from the ground and was pulled into your body by feather stroking, and that this Aurora Borealis energy would heal you." In his Essential Oils Integrative Medical Guide, Dr. Young writes that the Lakota who were ill would stand facing the Lights, holding out their hands and deeply inhaling the air that was charged with healing energy from the Aurora Borealis.

"My People would do this for several hours to several days with different shamans working on the sick individual. The healing energy from the Lights would also enter the shaman and pass through his/her hands into the person who was ill," Jeffrey explained. "And they did other things as well. They would 'feather' stroke the entire body, up and down, sideways, with their fingertips, both front and back." Jeff sat up and showed me. He used such a light touch that his fingers almost didn't touch my skin at all; it was truly an "energy process." "Occasionally they would use feathers, too. Especially when they could not go across the Canadian border to the Northern Lights."

Dr. Young has written much the same thing: Once the Lakota were restricted to their reservations in the United States, they practiced the feathering in other ways to spread the healing energy throughout the body. Jeffrey has been a massage therapist for many years, and is well known in Paducah. While in the Air Force, he also worked in hospitals as a Medical Illustrator, long before we had digital imaging available. The surgeons relied on his accurate medical drawings to visualize the necessary anatomy. These days he uses his finely tuned visualization skills to make extraordinary art.

Acknowledgements

Many thanks to:

Paul Horn, for my first introduction to sound healing and its amazing effects on the spirit of sentient beings, as seen in the whales he serenaded in British Columbia.

Jonathan Goldman, one of the foremost Sound Healers on the planet. In the last decade, I have continually derived inspiration from the multitude of his works, ranging from books explaining theory of sound healing to numerous CDs from which to experience firsthand healing with vibration. He emphasizes the importance of toning from within (chanting) to heal the organs, as well as the role of Intention combined with sound Frequency to create healing in his core concept of Frequency + Intention = Healing.

John Beaulieu, wayfarer on the path of Sound Healing since the 1970s, for his clarification of the importance of musical intervals as they affect our thoughts and feelings.

Hans Cousto for calculating the planetary frequencies from Keppler's work in the first place, and making this information widely known to further the healing efforts and research of individual healers all over the planet.

Donna Carey and **Marjorie de Mynck** for their groundbreaking work in creating Acutonics®, a cohesive system in which to apply tuning forks to the Extraordinary Vessels of Chinese medicine, the storehouse of our life force.

Teaming with **MichelAngelo,** gifted astrologer and musician, in creating detailed discussions of these vibrational intervals and their effects based upon the involved planetary body. And **Jude and Paul Ponton,** seasoned health practitioners, for using the forks, chimes and gongs in their busy private teaching practice to refine and clarify their uses in healing. Thank you, **Ellen Franklin**, for your crucial role in developing the Acutonics® work!

Dr. Andrew Weil, visionary physician who embodies the best of what one's doctor should be like: approachable, warm, wise, and with a wonderful sense of humor. And thanks to all my mentors at the University of Arizona Fellowship in Integrative Medicine program (Victoria Maizes, Randy Horowitz, Tieraona Low Dog), for continually raising the bar of excellence in delivering "the best medicine" from whatever source it comes.

Jeffrey Yuen, 88th generation Taoist priest, from whom I learned much about the use of essential oils in the context of Chinese medicine energetics. His gentle nature and personification of "cultivating the healer within" have left a strong imprint on my practice of medicine. Whenever Jeffrey came to the West Coast to lecture on essential oils, I was certain to be in the audience.

Gary Young, a true Visionary of our age, for leading the way in the cultivation, harvesting and use of essential oils, the "Missing Link" in the medicine of today and the future. We are probably too close to the ongoing accomplishments of his life to fully appreciate their enormity. Vibrational Raindrop Technique epitomizes the inspired application and anointing of aromatic frequencies to the body in our quest for returning to our original state of perfection as created by the Creator.

David and Lee Stewart, who tenaciously crafted the program for CARE (Center for Aromatherapy Research and Education), making the study of the chemistry of essential oils truly simple and a joy to pursue, as well as bringing Vibrational Raindrop Technique alive for me and a springboard from which to personalize and enhance its application in my professional practice as a physician.

As I contemplate the great minds and spirits of those persons mentioned herein, as well as the amazing times in which we live, I am very nearly overwhelmed at the beauty and precision of our Universe, and so much of it yet to be "discovered."

I can think of no greater past-time than this: to seek out evidence of the Divine Plan in every molecule around us. And on a more mundane, yet essential, level, I also want to thank all of those who found typos and made suggestions for improvements from the 1st edition of this book, and a special thanks goes to three CARE Instructors who have been teaching Vibrational Raindrop for some time now, viz. Joanna Barrett, Michelle Truman, and Bernadette Williams, for carefully and meticulously proofing the revised text before it went to press for the 2nd Edition.

Christi Bonds-Garrett, M.D.
Paducah, Kentucky

Table of Contents

Foreword

Vibrational Raindrop Technique originated in the 1980s through the research and practice of D. Gary Young. During its more than twenty-year history, it has undergone many refinements, changes, and variations.

Many of these modifications came as a consequence of the thousands taught by Gary Young over the years who added their own variations according to the perceived needs of their clients in their home areas. As a result, today there are literally hundreds of versions of Vibrational Raindrop Technique seen, taught, and practiced around the world.

Many of the different versions of Raindrop that exist today actually originated from Gary Young, himself, who customarily demonstrates different ways of doing Raindrop with every seminar he teaches. His stated reason for changing things with each demonstration is to customize and adapt the procedure according to the needs of the client upon whom he is working at the time.

However, the core of the Vibrational Raindrop Technique has remained relatively constant throughout the years in that the same suite of seven single oils and two blends are almost always used. Thus, the blends of Valor and AromaSeiz are always used, as well as the seven single species, namely, Oregano, Thyme, Wintergreen (or Birch), Basil, Marjoram, Cypress, and Peppermint. In addition, the means of applying the oils in Raindrop has also remained almost the same since the beginning, consisting of Vitaflex and other simple Vibrational Raindrop Techniques of applying fingers and hands to the feet and back.

Now Dr. Christi Bonds-Garrett has taken Raindrop Vibrational Raindrop Technique to another level. She hasn't changed the basic way of doing Raindrop. She consistently practices the version of Raindrop taught by D. Gary Young at a Young Living Training Workshop in Dallas, Texas, in January 2000.

There were more than 1000 participants who came from all over the world to learn Raindrop from Gary at that Seminar. Gary demonstrated Raindrop twice on two people in succession, with cameras rolling, indicating that this was to be his best and final version and that it would be published by Young Living as a VHS Video. (However, that Raindrop Video was never produced and Gary never taught it exactly like that again at any Young Living Training.)

Many, who have learned and done more than one version of Raindrop, themselves, and who have also practiced the version taught in Dallas in 2000, have concluded from their experiences that the way Gary taught Raindrop in that Dallas Seminar is one of his most effective versions. The Center for Aromatherapy Research and Education (CARE) has also come to that conclusion and has preserved Gary's original "Dallas" version of Raindrop since its founding in 2001. CARE Instructors continue to teach Raindrop that way to this day.

The version of Raindrop upon which this book is based is the one Gary taught in Dallas in 2000. It is also the one taught by CARE. It is referred to here as the "Classic Raindrop." The additional oils, outside of the nine oils of the original Raindrop, are also Gary Young's ideas. These are given on p. 299 of the 4th edition of the Essential Oils Desk Reference (EODR). However, these oils are only listed there, while their sequence and manner of use are not given. It was Dr. Bonds-Garrett who researched their various chemistries and vibrational characteristics to create the protocols for their applications, as presented in this book.

Dr. Bonds-Garrett is a medical doctor with certifications, internships, and residencies in psychiatry and family practice. She has also been a licensed homeopathic physician and is a practitioner of Chinese herbal medicine and reflexology. In addition, she is a Fully Certified CARE Instructor and well experienced with the applications of essential oils in her years of clinical practice.

No one could be more qualified to develop Raindrop and bring it to new levels than Dr. Christi Bonds-Garrett.

What you have in this book is a gift of twelve types of Vibrational Raindrop Technical, all based on the Classical Version, that address specific systems of the body. These twelve Raindrop protocols, originated and researched by Christi, use different assortments of oils for each application. These protocols also employ the frequencies and vibrations of tuning forks that resonate with your body's systems and stimulate their healing and balance. Through this book you now have a way to apply healing vibrations from two sources: 1. From the intrinsically high frequencies of essential oils; and 2. From actual vibrations of physical sound through tuning forks. Combining the two modalities, Dr. Bonds-Garrett has discovered and developed a set of powerful and new therapeutic protocols to address every body system in specific, targeted terms. Thus, the name "Vibrational Raindrop Technique."

In this book, Dr. Bonds-Garrett provides you with ten different Vibrational Raindrop Protocols. Starting with the 1. Classical Raindrop, fortified by tuning forks, she presents and explains Vibrational Raindrop Techniques for 2. Brain, 3. Colon & Digestion, 4. Heart & Circulation, 5. Hormone Balance for Women, 6. Hormone Balance for Men, 7. Joints & Bones, 8. Liver, 9. Lungs, 10. Longevity, 11. Metabolic Essentials, and 12. Bible Oils. Whatever your needs, Christi has exactly the Raindrop that would be best for you. All we can say is, Thank You, Doctor Christi. This work has been a labor of love on your part and now that love is going out to bless the world through this book. David Stewart, Ph.D., D.N.M. Marble Hill, Missouri

Introduction

As I sit here on a winter's day looking out over snow-covered fields from my view high above in the top floor of our Bird Wing, melodic strains of Jonathan Goldman's Celestial Reiki II fill the air, waxing and waning in volume and intensity.

My usually ebullient and frisky parrots are seemingly mesmerized by this music, eyes closed shut and heads wanting to tuck under their wings. It is still morning, and this is their time of usual greatest activity. But obviously the calming effect of Jonathan's music is more powerful than the time of day.

In one way or another, I have been involved with sound and essential oils for more than 20 years. I suppose I first noticed the amazing effects of sound frequencies on animals while I was previewing Andrew Weil and Kimba Arem's CD called Self-Healing with Sound and Music. Working at the computer on another project with a deadline, I had slipped the CD into the computer's player, thinking I would accomplish two projects at the same time. Apollo, my African Grey parrot, was climbing all over my lap, trying to chew the computer keyboard, and generally making a pest of himself. The moment the first notes of Track One were played, Apollo went into a trance state: he became absolutely still, cocked his head to the side, and appeared to be lost in his thoughts as he listened to the music of didgeridoos and singing bowls. This particular CD is composed of music and sounds that move from a higher frequency of Beta brainwave activity through Alpha and Theta down to Delta, and has been used successfully for insomnia by many of my patients.

At the time, I was beginning a two-year Fellowship in Integrative Medicine at the University of Arizona under the guidance of Dr. Andrew Weil, the Harvard-trained physician whose face on book and magazine covers is a familiar site to most Americans. Indeed, Time Magazine named him one of the 25 most influential Americans in 1997 and one of the 100 most influential people in the world in 2005. Always at the forefront of integrating the best and most diverse medicine out there, Dr. Weil has created a program at the University of Arizona to educate western trained physicians in the rapidly growing field known as Integrative Medicine (IM). His Arizona Center for Integrative Medicine defines IM as "healing-oriented medicine" that takes account of the whole person (body, mind, and spirit), including all aspects of lifestyle. It emphasizes the therapeutic relationship and makes use of all appropriate therapies, both conventional and alternative.

There is a lot of information packed into that definition, which describes a fundamental shift in how we practitioners of "western medicine" should deliver healthcare. It acknowledges the necessary partnership between patient and practitioner in healing-oriented medical care, and is predicated on a foundation that includes all the many factors influencing our states of health such as mind, body, spirit—and community.

As I sit here in the Bird Wing today listening to Celestial Reiki II, I am also reminded of the flute music of Paul Horn, which I first heard in the early 1970s. In 1968 Paul, a jazz musician and musical pioneer, was in India filming a documentary. One dark night, he took his flute into the dome of the Taj Mahal and played to the stars, haunting melodies of exquisite joy. Over the years, I listened to his music frequently, and it never failed to transport me to a place of inspiration and healing.

A few years later I heard that Paul would be appearing in a small theater in Portland, Oregon. I made certain to be there. Rather than performing his Taj Mahal music, however, he presented a show about playing the flute to killer whales in British Columbia! The whales came to him at poolside, intently listening with their faces poking out of the water, leaning on the rim of the pool, nuzzling him and his flute, and eventually answering his music with their own. Most of us left the little theater that magical evening shaking our heads in wonderment, little appreciating the larger healing message that Paul was revealing to us. The importance of sound, vibration, frequency, intention, shape/form and their interrelatedness become more obvious on a daily basis. Jonathan Goldman, a respected sound healer for decades, is well-known for his equation, "frequency + intention = healing." Throughout this book I will refer to this equation, substituting my own preferred methods of creating frequency and intention to obtain the desired outcome of healing.

Dr. Weil teaches, "Good medicine is based in good science. It is inquiry-driven and open to new paradigms." We will explore the rapidly emerging paradigm of frequency-based medicine, whether that frequency comes from the sound of tuning forks, the substance of essential oils, or other modalities which are composed of frequencies. Which, when you think about it, is just about everything!

January 2011
Paducah, Kentucky

Introduction to the Second Edition

Since the publication of the first edition of Vibrational Raindrop Technique in March 2011, I have been overwhelmed with questions about the many types of tuning forks available, and how they differ from the ones I use with Vibrational Raindrop Technique (VRT). Indeed, my choice of planetary frequencies was a difficult one, and was made only after long deliberation and study of the other major systems currently available. In this second edition, I have added more about the origin of the planetary frequencies and their traditional meanings in mythology.

I have created multiple versions of Vibrational Raindrop Technique using the "Twelve Oils of Ancient Scripture" Kit from Young Living® Essential Oils, and included my favorite one in this edition. The oils are applied in a meaningful anointing sequence to follow the New Testament life of Christ. Three Wise Men® is used in place of Valor® for the opening balancing blend. Some of the thicker or hotter oils (onycha, myrrh, cassia and galbanum) are applied on specific Neuro-Endocrine Centers along the spine, prior to "raindropping" a second major oil. The first oil is used as a catalyst to open the particular Center, thus strengthening the intention of the second raindropped oil. For those who are well-versed in both the Old and New Testaments, I invite you to create other sequences of anointing with these healing oils!

I've also included some advanced Vibrational Raindrop Techniques: explanations of different methods of using different octaves of forks (low and non-weighted forks); a timely VRT "Metabolic Essentials" protocol that uses YLEO's Slique Essence blend; and the use of Gem Tip Om tuning forks. In order to fully explain how these different octaves are effective, it will be necessary to briefly discuss Energy Anatomy including Neuro-Endocrine Centers (Chakras).

April 2012
Paducah, Kentucky

Introduction to the Third Edition

It is with much gratitude that I see a Third Edition of Vibrational Raindrop Technique come to press. What began in 2011 as a small project in tribute to the genius of Dr. D. Gary Young has developed a robust life of its own, ever growing all over the planet. It now includes three different frequency systems of tuning forks: the original Planetary plus the expanded Sacred Solfeggio, and finally a Pythagorean system.

The Planetary frequencies, the Sacred Solfeggio frequencies and the Pythagorean frequencies form a trinity of a whole system. The Sacred Solfeggio frequencies work on the Microcosmic, personal level and can take us to the inner universe deep within ourselves. With the linking frequencies of the Pythagorean (Mesocosmic) frequencies, they assist us to connect to the Macrocosmic level of the Planetary frequencies, which guide us to find our place in the outer universe.

Disease manifests in the physical, Newtonian world in which we live. But its root causes are in the nonphysical, Quantum world. The Pythagorean frequencies (body) are the link between the Sacred Solfeggio (mind) and the Planetary (spirit). Combining these sacred frequencies with the healing properties of essential oils, and applying them to ancient Chinese acupuncture points brings together multiple healing modalities, each with its own powerful morphic field. All together they bring balance to the orbits of our lives.

In the last few years, we have discovered that *VIBRATIONAL* Raindrop Technique supports the Human Energy Field: the Biofield, in modern terminology. As such, it is more appropriate to use less essential oil when using these vibrational modalities in conjunction with Raindrop Technique. In fact, we are actually working in the realm of Subtle Aromatherapy when our intention is to support the Biofield, and this means using essentials in nonphysical ways. The oils truly become the carriers of our Intention. According to the Arndt-Schultz Law, weak concentrations of biological agents stimulate physiological activity, medium concentrations of agents depress physiological activity, while large concentrations halt physiological activity.

For that reason, we use less essential oil in VRT: usually 1-2 drops is sufficient when used in combination with tuning forks.

We may use even less oil (1 drop) when used in combination with multiple modalities (tuning forks, color, etc.). Raindrop a carrier oil such as V-6 to the spine prior to raindropping essential oils. Not only does this carrier oil provide for proper "glide" of the tuning fork along the huato jiaji or muscle bands, it also provides the biofield and body more support to find its own innate wisdom to heal.

Hands-on training may be done with the excellent AromaSounds Coaches (www.AromaSounds.com), and Certification as a VRT Specialist (a form of Spiritual Healing) may be obtained through the National Therapies Certification Board (ntcb.org). I continue to offer new, innovative classes several times per year in historic LowerTown Arts District of Paducah, Kentucky. See you there!

May 2015

What is Vibrational Raindrop Technique (VRT)?

Vibrational Raindrop Technique (VRT) uses tuning forks to add the power of vibration to the healing energy of essential oils in Vibrational Raindrop Technique. In VRT, tuning forks are used in pairs to create "Intervals" of sound, starting with a Unison (two forks at the same frequency) and including a 2nd, 3rd, 4th, 5th, 6th, 7th, and Octave (two forks at a 2:1 frequency). Each of these vibrational/musical intervals has traditional qualities associated with it, which are then combined with essential oils at each step of Vibrational Raindrop Technique. For instance, a Perfect 5th interval (ratio of 2:3) is created when using the Om fork (136.10 Hz) with the Neptune fork (211.44 Hz). This interval balances the Autonomic Nervous System as these forks are applied to the Huato Jiaji points along the spine, and is specific for scoliosis (according to Acutonics).

Other essential oils can be used in place of the traditional Raindrop oils, making Vibrational Raindrop Technique useful for body systems like the Brain, the Liver, Joints and Hormones. The essential oil protocols in this book are based on the Wheel of suggested oils for these systems on page 299 of the 4th Edition of the Essential Oils Desk Reference (EODR). Valor®, Oregano and Thyme remain in every system's protocol, but the other six oils vary according to the body system.

In this book, we will discuss frequency/vibration and its effect on living systems in general, then get into the specific frequency intervals with their associated energetic effects.

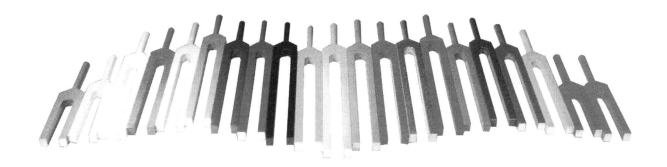

What is Raindrop Technique?

Vibrational Raindrop Technique uses tuning forks to add the power of vibration to Raindrop Technique, which was developed by Dr. Gary Young during the 1980s based on his knowledge of essential oils' antimicrobial effects coupled with the generation of electrical energy in the body. Raindrop Technique is a method of applying therapeutic grade essential oils to the feet and back/spine using special techniques such as Vitaflex ("vitality through the reflexes"), effleurage (feathered finger stroking), and dropping the oils in "raindrop" fashion onto the back.

With Vitaflex, electrical energy is generated with the pressure of the pad of the fingers on the skin. It is then released along nerve pathways when the electrical circuit is broken as the finger tips roll over onto the fingernail. In Raindrop Technique, essential oils are applied with Vitaflex onto spine reflex points on the soles of the feet. Thumb Vitaflex technique is also applied along the spine.

The French model for aromatherapy is followed in VRT, using undiluted essential oils. Some of the more well-known practitioners of the French model in the last 40 years include Rene Gattefosse, PhD, Jean Valnet, MD, Jean-Claude Lapraz, MD, Kurt Schnaubelt, PhD, and Daniel Penoel, MD. Rupert Sheldrake, well-known evolutionary biologist, coined the term "morphogenetic field" in the 1980s to describe a hypothesis of formative causation in his book *A New Science of Life*. He asked the question, why do plants and other biological entities develop the way they do? And what makes them change their patterns, as a whole, of genes and DNA was not enough to explain it. He proposed the idea that biological organization depends on "fields," which have been variously called biological fields, developmental fields, or "morphogenetic fields." These fields impose patterns on otherwise random patterns of activity.

Morphogenetic fields evolve over time; they are not fixed. Sheldrake compares the different morphic fields of Afghan hounds and poodles, which have a common ancestor in the wolf. These fields are inherited through an inherent memory in their genes, as well as a non-local resonance which he calls "morphic resonance." The "hundredth monkey effect" is cited as an example where a learned behavior spreads spontaneously from one group of monkeys to all related monkeys. It occurs when a critical number is reached who have learned the particular behavior. Sheldrake contends that a phenomenon like the "hundredth monkey effect" would be evidence of morphic fields bringing about non-local effects in consciousness and learning.

In Sheldrake's book The Presence of the Past, he further develops the idea of morphic fields to include any organizing fields of animal and human behavior, of social and cultural systems, and of mental activity, since they all contain inherent memory which evolves over time. In my opinion, Raindrop Technique is a new morphic field which is evolving through morphic resonance over time. More will be written about this concept in my book, *Raindrop Harmonics*.

About Essential Oils

Essential Oils are the life blood of a plant, and are vital to the life of the plant. Most of the time they are produced by steam distillation. They are composed of hundreds of compounds that are individually very tiny, usually much smaller than 300 atomic mass units (amu or daltons). It is because of this small size that the molecules of essential oils are aromatic; they can diffuse in the air and stimulate our sense of smell through Cranial Nerve 1, which goes directly to the limbic system and affects our emotions.

Any single essential oil may have hundreds of different molecules. Orange oil (citrus sinensis) contains 34 alcohols, 30 esters, 20 aldehydes, 14 ketones, 10 carboxylic acids, and 36 varieties of terpenes including mono-, sesqui-, di- and tetraterpenes! Since no essential oil has been completely analyzed, this analysis of orange oil cannot be considered complete.

Essential oils perform many functions in plants as well as in people: they assist metabolism, act as types of hormones and ligands, fight off infections by viruses, bacteria, parasites and fungi, and always work towards maintaining balance, or homeostasis, within the plant or person.

An essential oil must be distilled by therapeutic grade standards in order to extract an oil that is as close to nature as possible. Distillation must be done slowly, at low pressure, and at a relatively low temperature. The chemical profile of the primary constituents must fall within or *exceed* the parameters and standards of AFNOR (Association Francaise de Normalization) and/or ISO (International Standards Organization). While the AFNOR standard is actually only a perfume and food grade standard, at least it is a beginning step to identify minimal profiles of essential oils. There are no therapeutic grade standards in North America yet.

Therapeutic grade essential oils are the only oils that are safe to use in a therapeutic manner. Unfortunately, over 90% of the essential oils produced today are for the perfume and food industries and would not be good choices to use in Vibrational Raindrop Technique. While there are other sources of therapeutic grade essential oils, this book advises the reader to use only Young Living essential oils for Vibrational Raindrop Technique.

Vegetable oils (or "fatty acids" to chemists) come from the seeds of plants, are much larger than essential oils, and subsequently do not have much aroma. They are not essential to the life of the plant but instead provide nourishment to new seedlings. They can be used to slow down the absorption into the skin of an essential oil (such as using V-6 in Raindrop), or as a carrier for more dilute blends of essential oils (such as Ortho-Ease in Raindrop). In VRT, we use V-6, a vegetable oil blend, to "raindrop" before adding the essential oils since the additional vibrational modalities intensify the effects of the essential oils.

Chinese Medicine and Essential Oils

I have included some basic information on the use of the oils according to Chinese medicine interpretation since I am always thinking in that medical model as well. Chinese medical theory has a logical, codified system for the diagnosis and treatment of disease. Blood, Qi, and Yin/Yang are at the foundation of this system with Yin and Yang manifesting pathologically in concepts of cold and hot, deficiency and excess, damp and dry. They generally relate to two opposites that need to be held in balance. "Qi" is simply translated as "life force" or as "energy." Essential oils address three distinct constitutional levels described by Chinese medicine: the wei (protective meridians), ying (the twelve regular meridians and divergent meridians) and yuan (eight ancestral meridians, or extraordinary vessels).

Traditional Chinese Medicine (TCM) encompasses a comprehensive medical theory as well as an extensive pharmacopoeia which is organized into 24 categories by action. Each herb is explained through its energetics as well as its actions and the particular organ meridian it affects. According to Chinese herbal energetics, some herbs have ascending actions, while others descend; some invigorate while others sedate. Some herbs move to the body's surface or the extremities, while others penetrate deeply to affect organ functioning. At the root of it all is the most fundamental Kidney Qi: that which provides us with vitality and ensures proper function of all other organs.

Sound, Frequency and Form

Sound is the primary creative force in the universe! Sound came first, with all of creation following. Many cultures concur with this thought: In the book of Genesis from the Old Testament, one of the first statements is, "And God said, 'Let there be light; and there was light'." (Genesis 1:3) God speaks the name "Light" and through this creates light. Sound came before Light. "And the Spirit of God moved upon the face of the waters" before God spoke light into being. (Genesis 1:2)

In the Gospel according to John in the New Testament, it is written, "In the beginning was the Word, and the Word was with God, and the Word was God." (John 1:1) Words come from sound, and the word/sound was in the beginning. Light again comes after sound: "In him was life; and the life was the light of men." (John 1:4)

According to Jonathan Goldman, the ancient Egyptians believed that their god Thoth would speak the name of an object, and it would come into Being. In the Vedas, it says, "In the beginning was Brahman with whom was the Word." Spider Woman of the Hopi legends sang the song of creation over the inanimate forms on earth, bringing them to life. In the Popul Vuh in Mayan tradition, the first people are given life by the power of the voice. Similar legends exist in the Australian Aboriginal traditions, Polynesia and the Far East, as well as many African tribes. They all agree that the origin of the world came through Sound.

Sound is energy in wave form which is measured in amplitudes and cycles per second, its frequency. Everything is in a state of vibration, and therefore everything can be considered as a form of sound. As the ancient Sanskrit saying goes, "Nada Brahma," or "the world is sound." Sound is synonymous with God, so "the world is sound, and sound is Brahma/ God." To Joachim Berendt, this means that the world vibrates in harmonic

proportions, which he discusses at great length in his book, *The World is Sound: Nada Brahma.*

In quantum physics, terms such as "everything is sound" relate to electrons moving around the nucleus of an atom, and planets moving around the star of their galaxy, while galaxies move around a larger Source.

We hear sound in the range from 20 to 20,000 cps, or Hertz (named after the German physicist who first discovered radio waves, Heinrich Rudolph Hertz, 1857-1894). We can also "feel" very low frequencies even when we can barely hear them. Our range of hearing diminishes as we age, with a higher range of hearing in our youth. Mice have an extremely high range of hearing and can hear sound waves up to 100,000 cps, while dolphins have a range up to 180,000 cps! Even though we cannot hear that range of frequencies, it still exists and our bodies absorb and respond to it. Other animals are able to hear this range and can sound it. The faster the frequency, the higher the sound (treble), and the slower the frequency, the lower the sound (bass).

Sound creates form. One of the most well-known scientists to explore this idea was Dr. Hans Jenny, who put different substances (such as lycopodium powder) on a plate and vibrated the plate with varying frequencies of sound. The inert substance would spring to life into symmetrical shapes and designs. He also discovered that each organ of the body makes sound at specific frequencies. While they cannot be heard by the human ear, these sonic vibrations are measureable.

He and a colleague in England, Dr. Peter Manners, calculated what these frequencies are. If diseased, an organ ceased emitting its key note. But when its key note was aimed at it, the diseased organ was restored to health: the diseased organs were brought back to health through resonance with a healthy frequency. Dr. Jenny's work is documented in his book, *Cymatics*, and his DVDs showing the shifts in patterns are available as well.

Other scientists have explored the effects of sounds on matter, and have found that specific sounds used in meditation create specific shapes. One of the most amazing examples occurred when a Buddhist monk sounded "Om" into a tonoscope, and the mandala associated with Om was created by the tonoscope! This mandala consists of multiple overlapping triangles pointing up and down, just like the symbol associated with the 6th chakra, or energy center. Sound and form are interrelated. According to Steven Halpern, "Sound is a carrier wave of consciousness."

While filming Journey Inside Tibet in its highlands, Paul Horn paused for a moment in the vast empty terrain and said, "you hear that stillness?... It's silence... but it's filled with potential." Like breathing with its phases of exhalation and inhalation, as well as communing with the Divine via the two phases of prayer and meditation, Sound healing has phases of audible sound and echo, or silence. This is the Still Point, from which all potential arises. If you look at the close-up films of Dr. Jenny's tonometer while it makes geometric shapes, you will notice that the grains of powder are always moving toward the place of zero movement, or the node. The node attracts the particles of powder, which keeps the overall pattern congruent and orderly. As the tone/vibration into the tonometer is changed, the powder pauses in a still point, recognizes the new tone, and moves into the new form/pattern. As it changes form, there is a period of disorder, or chaos. The old form must break down in order for the new form to take shape.

Belgian scientist Ilya Prigogine described this phenomenon of order from chaos with his Theory of Dissipative Structures for which he was awarded the Nobel prize in 1977. It is in the nature of living biological systems to dissipate energy and move towards internal dissonance over time. As we move further away from equilibrium/balance, a point is reached where the internal "wobble" is so great that the system breaks down into chaos, or disease. This wobble and eventual chaos is a signal that something is changing inside, or is trying to change. We need to shift into "neutral" or a Still Point, in order to facilitate the change. The more we resist, the more difficult it is to make the change with grace. Overt chaos, or disease, can be the result.

Let's revisit the Old Testament. In Genesis, Chapter One, it says, "In the beginning God created the heaven and the earth. And the earth was without form, and void; and darkness was upon the face of the deep." Here was the moment of chaos with the potential for a shift into a greater reality. "And God said, Let there be light and there was light." God spoke/sounded/vibrated His creation into being. Before every act of creation, at least seven more times, we find that God spoke things into being: "And God said..."

How do we assist this Still Point within us to be found? It is certainly there; God has placed it there. It is a matter of frequency tuning, and this can be done with tuning forks as well as sound or other vibrational tools, such as essential oils. Every object has a natural frequency, which is the fundamental frequency at which it vibrates. For optimal function, objects need to be within their natural vibration, but sometimes they shift out into an unnatural resonance. We can assist the body to find its natural and perfect resonances by entraining it with tuning fork vibrations as well as coupling it with the intention inherent in essential oils. The ability of essential oils to go deep within the body, virtually any and everywhere, is a method to take the vibrational frequencies within.

Essential Oils & Intention

Every essential oil is composed of a variety of molecular components, and each of these components has a frequency associated with it. The larger the molecule is, the more complex and the greater the spectrum of frequencies. These frequencies are usually measured in mega-megahertz and higher. A megahertz (Mhz) vibrates at a rate of one million times per second (106 Hz), and a mega-megahertz (MMhz) vibrates at a trillion times per second (1012)! Double bonds between carbon atoms vibrate between 49-68 MMhz, double bonds between carbon and oxygen atoms between 51-53 MMhz, and single bonds between carbon and oxygen between 30-39 MMhz. Conclusion: **There is a lot of potential energy "zipped" into molecules of essential oils!**

How do we tap into this incredible source of energy? The body has a natural intelligence and ability to access these vibrational qualities of essential oils, much like playing the keys on a piano which sets vibrating strings in motion. In modern "String Theory" the entire universe is conceived as being composed of tones like a vibrating violin string, and a pluck of a string at one point will affect all the other strings in various degrees.

A little explanation is needed here before we talk about the "useable" frequency of a molecule of essential oil. When we hear the note of C in a Just scale, we are hearing 256 Hz. Depending on what instrument played that note, it will sound a little different, and the identity of the instrument will be readily known. This is because of "harmonics"—the additional tones/pitches that are sent out when an instrument plays a note. These are the "color" of sound, technically known as timbre.

If two slightly different frequencies are played simultaneously, they can reinforce one another and more importantly, they can cancel out each other, leaving a smaller and more manageable frequency. What is left is the difference in frequency between the two notes. For instance, two frequencies such as 256 Hz and 260 Hz could be played, and produce a frequency as low as 10 Hz or less. This is called a "beat frequency." In terms of essential oils with many molecules in the mega-megahertz range, they can combine within the single oil to create a net beat frequency in the lower megahertz range. These lower beat frequencies can act as the Fundamental in a harmonic group.

It is critical to note that these healing properties of essential oils apply only to pure, therapeutic grade oils! Their molecules form a coherent and harmonious family designed to heal us. If the oil is modified in any way (removing some constituents, adding synthetic ingredients, or adulterating it in other ways), it no longer is able to work in a coherent, functional way. Imagine having a perfectly trained orchestra performing a symphony, and a critical musician and instrument is replaced by a non-musical stranger who happens to be walking down the street. The entire orchestra will be disrupted and fall apart into dissonance.

Essential oils can also be affected by our thoughts. As described in the *Higleys' Reference Guide to Essential Oils,* Bruce Tainio in Washington was able to measure fundamental frequencies of people in various states of health as well as food, herbs and therapeutic grade essential oils. The healthy human ranges from 62-68 Mhz overall, fresh produce 10-15 Mhz, dry herbs 12-22 Mhz, processed/canned foods 0 Mhz, and therapeutic grade essential oils 52-320 Mhz. Rose has the highest frequency (320 Mhz) of single essential oils. But even more interesting is the effect that one's thoughts had on the oils. When the oils were subjected to negative thoughts, their frequencies decreased by 12 Mhz, and with positive thoughts they increased by 15 Mhz. **Oils can serve as a vehicle to amplify intention.**

Many have heard of the work of Dr. Masaru Emoto, the Japanese scientist who discovered that molecules of water are affected by our thoughts, words, and feelings. Originally conducting research into the measurement of wave fluctuations in water, he discovered that water has the ability to copy information.

With some perseverance Emoto was able to develop a method to photograph water crystals as they emerge from ice for 20–30 seconds while the temperature rises and the ice begins to melt.

He experimented with the effect of music on water, as well as words written on paper and wrapped around the water container. Water which was exposed to the music of Beethoven or Mozart showed bright, symmetrical forms, and the word "love" generated a complex and exquisite molecule. Angry words as well as exposure to microwaves and cell phones generated malformed crystals.

Photographs of the resulting crystal shapes should indeed give us each pause for thought. And since humans as well as the earth are composed mostly of water, the "Messages from Water" are profound in their applications to us. Essential oils, like water, have frequency and can carry intention. Since water is everywhere in our bodies, so, too, can essential oils access anywhere in the body. They have an innate wisdom that knows where to go and what to do to heal the human body. They also heal the emotions and spirit.

Intervals, Energetics, & Tuning Forks

In order to understand the energy behind the tuning forks, we need to learn a little about music theory.

An **interval** is the distance between two notes/tones/pitches. Two notes are harmonic if they are sounded at the same time, while they would be called melodic if sounded in succession. We always use two tuning forks at the same time in Vibrational Raindrop Technique, and thus are always working with harmonic musical intervals. Similarly, a **chord** is a set of three or more notes that is heard simultaneously.

There are seven pitches or tones in the Western **diatonic** musical scale: for example: A through G, which are the white keys on a piano. But there are 12 actual notes that divide an octave if you also include the black keys. When the 12 notes are played in succession from one tone to the octave above or below, it is called a **chromatic** scale. Five of the 12 notes fall between the seven main tones; these are the black keys (sharps and flats) on a piano. Each pitch of tempered chromatic scale is the same interval away from the previous pitch. A sharp raises the natural note, and a flat lowers the note.

INTERVALS

An **interval** is the sound that results when two tones/pitches are sounded at the same time. It is a point that results from the meeting of the two waves of two tones. Some intervals are naturally and traditionally pleasing to us: the Octave (2:1), 5ths (3:2) and 4ths (4:3), where the frequencies of the two notes are proportionately 2 to 1, 3 to 2, and 4 to 3, respectively. Thus, Middle C on the piano vibrates at 261.63 Hz while the note an octave below vibrates at half that rate, or 130.82 Hz, hence the 2:1 ratio of frequencies. Octaves, 5ths and 4ths are referred to as the "perfect intervals" in music because the

ratios of the two frequencies comprising these intervals are exact whole numbers.

These harmonic ratios were used to create architecture long ago, and the most beautiful temples in the ancient worlds of Athens, Rome and Egypt are based upon these proportions.

A proportion known as the Golden Section was extremely important to ancient architects, and architecture has been called "music frozen in time." It says that the ratio of the whole to the larger part is the same as the ratio of the larger part to the smaller part. These proportions are found in the human body, as well as plants, insects and animals. For instance, the thigh is to the calf as the arm is to the forearm, as the lower part of the body is to the upper with the navel as the dividing point. Musically, the Golden Section is found in the ratios of the Major 6th (3:5) and the minor 6th (5:8).

MUSIC IS MOVEMENT

The nature of music exists in movement. It starts from a specific point, then moves through different notes or intervals to create tension, and then releases the tension.

Consonance and dissonance arise when two notes are sounded together, creating an interval which is either pleasing and relaxing (**consonant**) or unstable, energetic and full of movement (**dissonant**). These are not absolute definitions since the response to an interval is highly subjective and related to cultural background.

For instance, in the past only a few overtones of a given fundamental were considered consonant: the unison, octave, 5th and 4th. In today's world, we experience most intervals as relatively consonant and pleasing. But the 2nds, 7ths and tritones (augmented 4ths) are the most dissonant and therefore full of tension. They can be used to generate a high state of energy and movement, and are critical for growth and evolution.

I wonder if you noticed that I slipped in another word in the previous paragraph without defining it? An *overtone* is any frequency higher than the fundamental tone. Together, they are called partials and create harmonics when their frequencies are whole number multiples of the fundamental. For instance, in our VRT system the fundamental is Om 136.10 Hz, so harmonic overtones would have frequencies in whole number multiples of Om, such as 272.20 Hz, 544.40 Hz, 1088.80 Hz, and on and on.

While overtones theoretically progress to infinity, we will hear them up to only about 20,000 Hz, or maybe not even that high depending upon your range of hearing. But remember: just because we cannot hear them, doesn't mean that they don't exist and don't have an effect! In VRT we also use lower multiples of the fundamental such as the Low Om tuning fork with a frequency of 68.05 Hz. It is this spectrum of tones that range from the fundamental tone up into kilohertz of cps that gives a sound its "color" or timbre, and allows it to be differentiated from other sources (instruments) of sound. Jonathan Goldman has an equation that relates frequency to healing:

Frequency + Intention = Healing

The intervals of the tuning forks represent the "Frequency" term, "Intention" is represented by the choice of the specific essential oil, and "Healing" is the desired outcome. Thus, this equation can be rewritten as:

Tuning Forks + Essential Oils = Desired Outcome

An interval's quality is determined by its relationship to the Fundamental tone within the system being used. Two of the most common systems of tuning forks on the market today are those relating to a Fundamental of a multiple of 8 Hz (a Just scale), and those relating to a Fundamental of 136.10 Hz, which is the sound of Om (the sound of an Earth year, or the time it takes Earth to travel through the four seasons around the sun). A third popular system is the Sacred Solfeggio, derived from the book of Numbers in the Old Testament.

In the first and most well-known VRT, I am using the planetary tuning forks according to Hans Cousto's calculations with the tuning fork of Om/136.10 Hz as the fundamental tone. Using the Om fork with the planetary tuning forks creates intervals, whose characteristics continue to be explored by Donna Carey, Ellen Franklin, and Acutonics® practitioners around the world. The second system of VRT uses the Sacred Solfeggio frequencies. And the third system of VRT uses a Pythagorean system of frequencies with C 126 Hz as the fundamental. Energetics involves study, applications, and research regarding the energetic effects and properties of various frequencies on the mind and body, particularly the planetary, terrestrial, and lunar frequencies as expressed through tuning forks.

Planetary Tuning Fork Intervals

The name of each tuning fork (e.g. "Jupiter" or "Mars") represents a specific pitch or frequency calculated from the revolutionary period around the sun of the heavenly body for which it is named. The forks, their frequencies and their names are based on the astronomical calculations of Johannes Kepler in the 1620s. See *Cosmic Octave* by Hans Cousto for additional discussion of Om and how the frequencies of the planetary forks are made audible.

Following are some of the possible intervals that can be used with their associated musical and planetary energetics. The name of the interval is given (e.g. Unison), then its ratio with Om (e.g. 1:1), then the name of the tuning fork to be used with Om to produce that interval.

Unison, 1:1

Om/Om — centering, rooting and grounding

Microtone

Interval that is less than an equally spaced semitone. The primary microtones in this geocentric system (using Om as the Fundamental) occur near the Unison. They are necessary to help us move away from grounding and center, to move away from a comfort zone in order to explore new possibilities and stimulate expansion and growth from within.

Om/Pluto — highly dissonant, penetrates deep into the body structure to a cellular level, unconscious and shadow-self level, breaks down resistance to change. Disharmony between notes creates desire for resolution.

Om/Mercury — creates a great deal of movement and dissonance; volatile, going "between the cracks."

Minor 2nd, 15:16

Om/Mars — harsh; carrier of considerable energetic potential, propels the mind, body and spirit into action with power and initiative to remove obstacles.

Om/Saturn — semitone and somewhat dissonant, supports the formation of new boundaries and structures. The Minor Second is the most dissonant of the intervals, and Om/Saturn is more dissonant than Om/ Mars. They both represent the applications of energy toward the manifestation of material form, in other words creating matter from spirit. Twin pillars of evolution on the material and spiritual planes.

Major 2nd, 9:8

Om/Chiron Healer or **Low Om/Low Chiron Healer** or **High Om/High Chiron Healer** — dense but warmer than the minor 2nd; allows access to deep wounds and scars of a physical, emotional, or spiritual nature to transform and repair. Occurs between consonant interval (3rd) and dissonant intervals (minor 2nd), and thus is the space between harmony and disharmony. Modern Classical music.

Major 3rd, 4:5

Om/Zodiac Platonic Earth – optimistic, happy; meditative, dispersive or dispelling effect, relieves mental stress, but is especially useful to relieve physical stress.

Perfect 4th, 3:4

Om/Jupiter – Perfect Fourth; pure, like church bells; stimulates growth, abundance and expansion. The Fourth is the geometric mean of an Octave.

Augmented 4th, 45:32

Om/Earth Day – Full of movement, intense propelling energy. Also considered to be a Diminished 5th. Three degrees above the tritone (physical midpoint of the octave) of 191.39. This interval has been called Crux Ansata, a transition point where spirit is redeemed from matter.

Minor 6th, 5:8 *See the 3 different Fork Combinations below*

The Fifth is the halfway point (harmonic mean) between octaves, a "point of release" from a particular paradigm. In the key of "C" this would be the notes C and G sounded together. In the key of Om, this would be Om and a frequency about 204.15 hz sounded together. Many planets create a variation of the "perfect 5th", and each has its own keynote qualities which relate to the planet involved.

The 5th interval is pure, like church bells (like the Perfect 4th). The 5th interval is associated with the nitrogen atom (Berendt) and stimulates nitric oxide release by an unknown mechanism (Beaulieu 2003). Beaulieu postulates that nitric oxide acts locally as a hormone and neurotransmitter, is antimicrobial, enhances the immune system, balances the heart, pituitary gland and sphenoid bone, balances the autonomic nervous system. It is said to enhance the mobility of joints, and relieve depression.

This interval is the foundation of Gregorian chant in which the first section of the choir sings the fundamental tone and another section sings at the Fifth Interval. Because of the resonance of European cathedrals, only one melody needs to be sung as it bounces back the harmony of the Fifth (known as the Hildegard Thumbprint after Hildegard von Bingen, the 12th century mystic, herbalist and musician).

Om/New Synodic Moon – calming, opening, the New Beginnings Fifth, dispersive for emotional issues.

Om/Uranus – a Perfect Fifth, could be called the Transformative Fifth; opens with the electrical charge of transformation, can shatter pre-existing conceptions and embodies the energy of freedom.

Om/Neptune – a near Perfect Fifth, aptly called the Visionary Fifth, opens and moves the visionary from transpersonal to transcendental, fulfills the yearning for connection with the Infinite.

Minor 6th, 5:8

Om/Venus – a mellow sense of longing; tonifies, nourishes beauty, harmony and creative passion but has a quality of inconstancy, desire and yearning for completion. Inversion of the Major Third (4th harmonic of overtone series). A Major Third plus a Minor Sixth creates an Octave.

Major 6th, 3:5

Om/Full Sidereal Moon – optimistic, less emotional than the Major 3rd; builds energy, brings a feeling of fullness, unveiling, and purification; the ultimate expression of Yin. Can bring a sense of magic and fulfillment; is rhythmic with a pull towards healing that allows one's potential to manifest. Known as the Golden Section, Divine Proportion, or Golden Mean.

Minor 7th, 5:9

L Om/Sun – full of tensions, initiative, empowerment, vitalizing and warm, with unconditional love and the ultimate expression of yang. An inversion of the Major 2nd, and the two intervals create an Octave.

Om/High Sun – a bit harsh but more distant and less emotional than the Major 2nd (its inversion).

Octave, 1:2

Low Om/Om – Perfect Octave, dreams come true; brings feelings of comfort, grounding and unity.

High Sun/Angelic Sun – very warming and energizing, bright sunshine on a cloudy day.

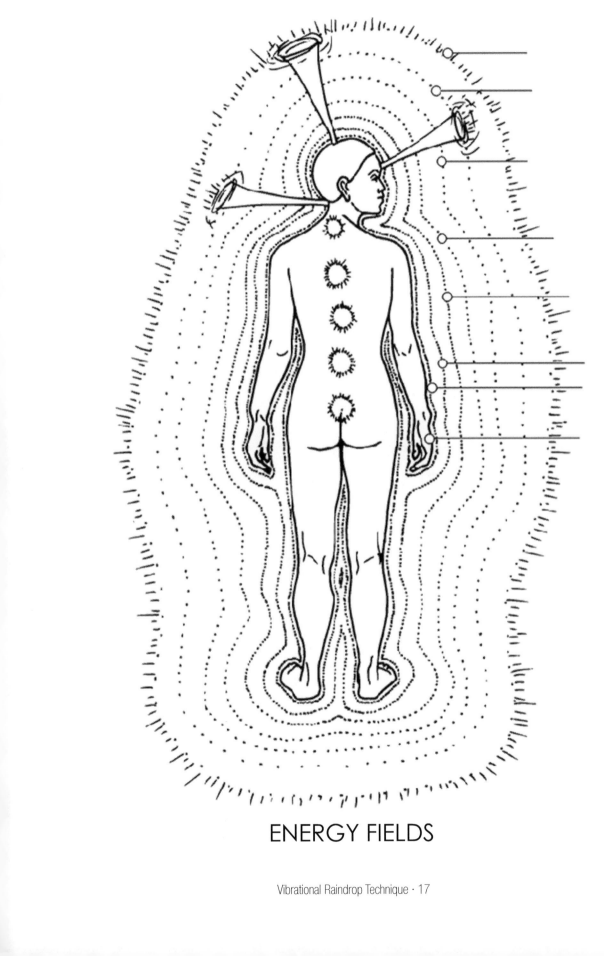

ENERGY FIELDS

Energy Anatomy

Here is a brief primer on Energy Anatomy, which you will need to be a little familiar with in order to do the Metabolic Essentials VRT. Energetic anatomy consists of two types of fields: "veritable" which can be measured, and "subtle" which cannot be measured. Measurable veritable fields include the physical fields of electromagnetism, Schumann waves, sound waves, magnetism, visible light and more. We make and feel both of these types of energy fields.

The subtle energy fields (the "Aura") are a continuation of the physical energy fields. Their effects can be seen, but they themselves cannot routinely be seen by all persons. They are connected to the physical fields of the body via the Neuro-Endocrine Centers (chakras) and along the Bonghan channels (acupuncture meridians), which have been found in lymphatics, veins and in web-like formation over organs. Our "vital force", or qi/chi, flows along these meridians as part of a larger energy matrix which links to the Central Nervous System (CNS).

Qi can be translated as energy, air, breath, vital breath, wind, vital essence, prana, and so on. It is in everything around and within us; it is the activating energy of the universe. While qi cannot be destroyed, it is often transformed and materializes in various forms and cycles of positive and negative (yang and yin) energy. Qi is the force that holds existence together, and does not belong to any single religious pathway.

The veritable (measurable) field will simply be called the Physical Body (Field 1). The Etheric Body (Field 2) connects the Physical Body to the lower subtle energy fields. Although there are many subtle energy fields, we will limit the discussion to six of them: the Lower Emotional body (Field 3), the Astral Body (Field 4), the Higher Emotional Body (Field 5), the Mental Body (Field 6), and the Spirit Body (Field 7). The Heart has an electromagnetic field that has its own unique qualities and identity.

Each of these fields is associated with a Neuro-Endocrine Center (Chakra), and there are various correlations with endocrine organs that are made in the many different systems of Chakra theory. What follows is a brief overview of the working model I use in my clinic.

Neuro-Endocrine Centers/ Chakras and Energy Fields

The **first** field, **Physical Body**, connects with the **Root Chakra** and the adrenal glands. It consists of the physical body plus the Physical-Etheric Body extends about one inch beyond the body. Sometimes it is visualized with a funnel shape that opens to earth. Some essential oils with an affinity for this level include Juniper, Geranium, Myrrh, Abundance, Grounding, and Valor. Its color is deep red, and the Garnet gemstone resonates with it. The Root Chakra is reached from the spine at GV-2. It has a relationship with the Crown Chakra.

The **second** field, **Etheric Body**, connects with the **Sacral Chakra** and the sexual glands (ovaries or testes), and the (Emotional) Etheric Body extends up to 4 inches above the Physical Body. This is the level at which the veritable field energies are transmitted into the Physical Body. Etheric energy connects with the Autonomic Nervous System (ANS), the Cerebro-Spinal Fluid (CSF), and the endocrine glands. This is the Body that is photographed with Kirlian photography. Some essential oils with an affinity for this level include Blue Spruce, Patchouli, Clary Sage, Highest Potential and Harmony. Its color is orange, and the Carnelian gemstone resonates with it. The Sacral Chakra is reached from the spine at GV-4 and anteriorly at CV-2. It has a relationship with the Throat Chakra since both of them are centers of creativity and expression.

The **third** field, **Lower Emotional Body**, connects with the **Solar Plexus Chakra** and the pancreas. It extends up to 12 inches above the Physical Body. This is where our fear-based limiting emotions are stored and where emotional release must take place before true healing will occur. The Solar Plexus Chakra is reached from the spine at GV-6 and anteriorly at CV-12. Some essential oils with an affinity for this level include Lemon, Release, Acceptance and Forgiveness. Its color is yellow, and the Citrine gemstone resonates with it. It has a relationship with the Brow Chakra.

The **fourth** field, **Astral Body,** connects with the **Heart Chakra** and the thymus gland. According to HeartMath Institute, the Heart is the most powerful generator of electromagnetic energy in the human body: its electric field is 60 times greater than the field generated by the brain. Even more stunning, the heart's magnetic field is more than 5,000 times greater than the brain's magnetic field! This magnetic field can be detected more than several feet away from the body. It is this powerful electromagnetic Heart Field that allows access to the "Zero Point Energy Field" of quantum physics, which is the lowest energy state of a field. Some people believe that this field is the one that connects the human being to the Divine. This is the field where we decide whether to experience Fear or Love in our daily lives. Some essential oils with an affinity for this level include Idaho Balsam Fir, Jasmine and Joy. Its color is green or pink, and both the Jade and the Rose Quartz gemstones resonate with it. The Heart Chakra is reached from the spine at GV-11 and anteriorly at CV-17.

The **fifth** field, **Higher Emotional Body**, connects with the **Throat Chakra** and the thyroid/parathyroid glands, and is generally thought to be up to 20 inches above the Physical Body. Emotions derived from love find their expression here. Some essential oils with an affinity for this level include Myrtle, Purification and Surrender. Its color is deep turquoise blue, and the Blue Topaz gemstone resonates with it. The Throat Chakra is reached from the spine at GV-14 and anteriorly at CV-22. It has a relationship with the Sacral Chakra since both of them are centers of creativity and expression.

The **sixth** field, the **Mental Body**, connects with the **Brow Chakra** and the pituitary gland. It is over 30 inches above the Physical Body. Thought Forms originate at this level, and this is where we visualize our future, either consciously or unconsciously. Some essential oils with an affinity for this level include Rosemary, Sandalwood, Awaken and Envision. Its color is deep blue to purple, and the Amethyst gemstone resonates with it. The Brow Chakra is reached from the base of the skull at GV-16 and anteriorly at Yin Tang (GV-24.5). The Locus Ceruleus can be activated through GV-16, Wind Mansion, and is an important balancing control center of the body, used in NeuroAuricular Technique.

And the **seventh** field, the **Spirit Body**, connects with the **Crown Chakra** and the pineal gland. This field is often seen as a funnel shape that opens to the heavens above the person's head. Some essential oils with an affinity for this level include Rose, Frankincense, and White Angelica. Its color is clear white, and the Clear Quartz gemstone resonates with it. The Crown Chakra is reached from the top of the head at GV-20. It has a relationship with the Root Chakra.

Applying tuning forks to access points of the Brow (GV-16) and Crown Chakras (GV-20) will activate the

"Crystal Palace" in the center of the brain, which includes the thalamus, hypothalamus, pineal and pituitary glands. The Crystal Palace has many nerve connections with the Locus Ceruleus ("blue spot") located in a part of the brain called the Pons.

Sometimes an acupoint is called a "micro-chakra" because they are energy vortices which provide access to the flow of qi (vital energy force).

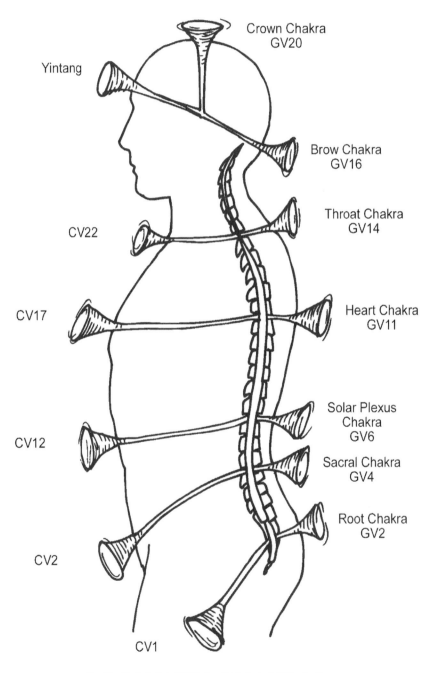

BODY WITH CHAKRAS

Chakras

ROOT CHAKRA – 1ST NEC

Rules: Physical Body

Body Part: Kidneys, Skeleton

Stone: Garnet

Emotions: Security, Support

Sense: Taste, mouth

Diseases: Arthritis, Osteoporosis

Endocrine: Adrenal Glands

Color: Deep Red

Archetype: Mother

Element: Earth

Access Points: GV2 or CV1

Essential Oils:

Singles: Black Pepper, Cardamom, Carrot Seed, Cedarwood, Citronella, Clary Sage, Clove, Cypress, Elemi, Frankincense, Geranium, Ginger Root, Golden Rod, Idaho Balsam Fir, Jasmine, Juniper, Melissa, Myrrh, Nutmeg, Oregano, Patchouli, Peppermint, Rosemary, Sage, Sandalwood, Vetiver, Ylang Ylang

Blends: Abundance, Dragon Time, EndoFlex, EnRGee, Forgiveness, Grounding, Highest Potential, Hope, Humility, Inner Child, Into the Future, Mister, Sclaressence, Release, SARA, Surrender, Traumalife, Valor

. . . .

SACRAL CHAKRA – 2ND NEC

Rules: Etheric Body

Body Part: Bladder

Stone: Carnelian

Emotions: Creativity, Abundance

Sense: Smell, Nose

Diseases: Reproductive problems, Sciatica

Endocrine: Sexual Glands

Color: Orange

Archetype: Empress

Element: Metal

Access Points: GV4 or CV2

Essential Oils:

Singles: Cinnamon Bark, Clary Sage, Coriander, Cypress, Fennel, Geranium, Grapefruit, Jasmine, Myrrh, Niaouli, Orange, Patchouli, Peppermint, Petitgrain, Pine Needles, Rose, Tangerine, Vetiver, Ylang Ylang

Blends: DiGize, Dragon Time, Harmony, Hope, Inner Child, Joy, Purification, Sensation

SOLAR PLEXUS CHAKRA – 3RD NEC

Rules: Lower Emotional Body

Body Part: Stomach, Liver, Gallbladder, Pancreas

Stone: Citrine

Emotions: Self-esteem, Personal Power

Sense: Hearing, Ear

Endocrine: Pancreas Gland

Color: Yellow

Archetype: Warrior

Element: Water

Access Points: GV6 or CV12

Diseases: Gastritis, Hepatitis, Pancreatitis, Diabetes

Essential Oils:

Singles: Cardamom, Carrot Seed, Cinnamon Bark, Coriander, Dill, Fennel, Ginger, Grapefruit, Idaha Balsam Fir, Juniper, Ledum, Lemon, Lemongrass, Marjoram, Oregano, Peppermint, Sandalwood, Spikenard, Thyme, Valerian Root, Vetiver, Wintergreen, Ylang Ylang

Blends: DiGize, Forgiveness, Gentle Baby, GLF, Gratitude, Highest Potential, Hope, Humility, Inner Child, Into the Future, Juva Cleanse, JuvaFlex, Peace & Calming, Purification, Release, SARA, Surrender, Thieves, Transformation, TraumaLife, Valor

. . . .

HEART CHAKRA – 4TH NEC

Rules: Astral Body

Body Part: Heart, Lungs, Circulation

Stone: Rose Quartz, Jade

Emotions: Love

Sense: Sound, Vibration

Endocrine: Thymus

Color: Rose or Green

Archetype: Lover

Element: Water

Access Points: GV11 or CV17

Diseases: Atherosclerosis, Myocardial Infarction, Emphysema, Arrhythmias

Essential Oils:

Singles: Bergamot, Black Pepper, Carrot Seed, Cinnamon Bark, Clove, Cypress, Eucalyptus, Frankincense, Helichrysum, Hyssop, Inula, Jasmine, Lavender, Marjoram, Melissa, Neroli, Nutmeg, Oregano, Ravensara, Rose, Sage, Sandalwood, Spikenard, Thyme, Yarrow, Ylang Ylang

Blends: Acceptance, Aromalife, Believe, Citrus Fresh, Forgiveness, Joy, Rutavala, Valor

THROAT CHAKRA – 5TH NEC

Rules: Upper Emotional Body

Body Part: Throat, Thyroid, Jaws, Mouth

Stone: Blue Topaz

Emotions: Creativity, Integrity

Sense: Hearing, Inner Ear

Endocrine: Thyroid

Color: Turquoise

Archetype: Artist

Element: Water

Access Points: GV14 or CV22

Diseases: Hypothyroid, Laryngitis, TMJ, Neck problems

Essential Oils:

Singles: Carrot Seed, Cypress, Frankincense, Geranium, German Chamomile, Lavender, Lemongrass, Myrrh, Myrtle, Peppermint, Roman Chamomile, Sandalwood, Spearmint, Spruce

Blends: Awaken, Believe, Deep Relief, EndoFlex, Envision, Inspiration, Surrender, Thieves, Transformation, Valor

⋯⋯⋯⋯⋯⋯⋯⋯⋯⋯⋯⋯⋯⋯⋯⋯⋯⋯⋯⋯⋯⋯

BROW CHAKRA – 6TH NEC

Rules: Mental Body

Body Part: Eyes, Locus Ceruleus

Stone: Amethyst

Emotions: Wisdom, Intuition

Sense: Sight, Eye

Endocrine: Pituitary

Color: Purple

Archetype: Wise One

Element: Wood

Access Points: GV16 or Yin Tang

Diseases: Migraine, Vision problems, Strokes, Brain diseases

Essential Oils:

Singles: Cedarwood, Clary Sage, Frankincense, Geranium, Helichrysum, Juniper, Lavender, Lemongrass, Linden Blossum, Myrtle, Oregano, Pine, Rose, Rosemary, Sandalwood, Spruce, Thyme

Blends: Awaken, Endoflex, Envision, Inspiration, Surrender, Transformation, Valor, Helichrysum italicum, Linden Blossom

CROWN CHAKRA – 7TH NEC

Rules: Spirit Body

Endocrine: Pineal

Body Part: Cerebral Cortex, Skin

Color: White

Stone: Clear Quartz

Archetype: Enlightened One

Emotions: Serenity, Grace

Element: Fire

Sense: Voice, Tongue

Access Points: GV20

Diseases: Epilepsy, Learning Disabilities, Nervous Disorders, Insomnia

Essential Oils:

Singles: Angelica Root, Basil, Elemi, Frankincense, Idaho Blue Spruce, Lavender, Myrrh, Petitgrain, Ravensara, Rosemary, Rosewood, Sandalwood, Spikenard, Vetiver

Blends: White Angelica

Microcosmic Orbit

Most of the acupoints that are used in Vibrational Raindrop Technique are found on what is known as the **"Microcosmic Orbit."** This orbit of energy is like a large reservoir that supplies nourishing qi to the body along the Governor Vessel and Conception Vessel, which are two of the Ancestral Channels. When there is lots of nourishing energy, these channels are able to supply the rest of the body via the 12 principal meridians. When there is a blockage in these two channels, there will be a problem in the body.

The Microcosmic Orbit follows the pathway of the Conception Vessel and Governor Vessel, circulating up the spine, over the head, and down the front to connect the two channels in the lower Dan Tien (the primary center of life force energy located deep behind the navel). Its free and open flowing is essential to health on all levels and in all Neuro-Endocrine Centers. Using tuning forks, vibration, and frequencies on some of its key points is fundamental to healing.

The Orbit begins in the lower Dan Tien, then moves out to the navel and down to CV-2 (Curved Bone) to CV-1 (Meeting of Yin) in the perineum, moves up the spine to GV-1 (Long Strong), then continues up to GV-4 (Life Gate), GV-6 (Spinal Center), GV-11 (Spirit Path), GV-16 (Wind Mansion), GV-20 (Hundred Convergences) on the crown of the head. At this point, it goes over the head down the forehead to GV-24.5 (Yin Tang), connects with the Conception Vessel and moves down to CV-22 (Heavenly Prominence), goes down to CV-17 (Chest Center), CV-12 (Central Venter), CV-8 (Spirit Gate) at the navel and moves back into the lower Dan Tien. As you can see, the path of the Microcosmic Orbit connects the access points of the Neuro-Endocrine Centers to one another.

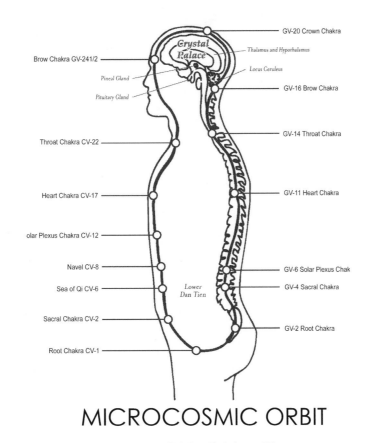

GV-20 Crown Chakra

Crystal Palace

Thalamus and Hypothalamus

Brow Chakra GV-241/2

Locus Ceruleus

Pineal Gland

GV-16 Brow Chakra

Pituitary Gland

GV-14 Throat Chakra

Throat Chakra CV-22

GV-11 Heart Chakra

Heart Chakra CV-17

olar Plexus Chakra CV-12

GV-6 Solar Plexus Chak

Navel CV-8

GV-4 Sacral Chakra

Sea of Qi CV-6

Lower Dan Tien

Sacral Chakra CV-2

GV-2 Root Chakra

Root Chakra CV-1

MICROCOSMIC ORBIT

Acupuncture Points for Tuning Forks

Acupuncture points are located in depressions between 1-5 sq.mm. in size that can be found by palpation, and frequently are sensitive. They have lowered resistance and high conductivity, and consist of a vertical column of loose connective tissue which contains a large lymphatic trunk, a large arteriole, and a satellite vein. These thin-walled vessels are surrounded by netlike arrangements of nerve fibers, both myelinated and unmyelinated. A high concentration of perineural cells and micro-vesicles can be found where the sympathetic nerve endings meet the walls of the vessels. Sometimes an acupoint is called a "micro-chakra" because they are energy vortices which provide access to the flow of qi (vital energy force).

KI 1 (Kidney 1, Gushing Spring) — on the sole at the border between the anterior and middle thirds of the foot, proximal to the second and third MTP joints; this point calms the spirit, revives consciousness and rescues Yang, and descends excess from the head.

CV 4 (Conception Vessel 4, Origin Pass) — Midline of the abdomen, 4 finger widths below the umbilicus; this point fortifies the Original Qi and Essence, and warms and benefits the Kidneys, Spleen, Bladder, Small Intestine, and Uterus.

CV 17 (Conception Vessel 17, Chest Center) — In the center of the chest, level with the 4th rib; this point unbinds the chest, opens energy, and allows for the heart beat and the lung breath to synchronize into a coherent pattern.

GV 2 (Governor Vessel 2, Low Back Shu) — at the base of the sacrum; this point benefits the lumbar region and legs, and dispels Wind Damp, First (Root) Neuro-Endocrine Center (Chakra).

GV 4 (Governor Vessel 4, Life Gate) — just below the 2nd lumbar vertebra; nourishes Source and Kidney energy, Second (Sacral) Neuro-Endocrine Center (Chakra)

GV 6 (Governor Vessel 6, Spinal Center) — below the 11th thoracic vertebra; benefits the spine, Third (Solar Plexus) Neuro-Endocrine Center (Chakra).

GV 11 (Governor Vessel 11, Spirit Path) — below the 5th thoracic vertebra; calms the spirit, gathers the Qi for the Lung and Heart, Fourth (Heart) Neuro-Endocrine Center (Chakra).

GV 14 (Governor Vessel 14, Great Hammer) — below the 7th cervical vertebra; meeting point of the Governor Vessel with the yang channels of the hand and foot; Fifth (Throat) Neuro-Endocrine Center (Chakra).

GV 16 (Governor Vessel 16, Wind Mansion) — in the depression directly below the occipital protuberance, 1 finger width above the middle of the natural hairline at the back of the head; this point calms the spirit, eliminates "wind", and benefits the head and neck; Sixth (Brow) Neuro-Endocrine Center (Chakra); access point to the Locus Ceruleus.

GV 20 (Governor Vessel 20, Hundred Convergences) — on the midline of the head, about 9 finger widths directly above the posterior hairline, on the midpoint of the line connecting the apices of the ears; this point benefits the brain and calms the spirit, benefits the head and sense organs, raises Yang and counters prolapse, and nourishes the sea of marrow (brain and spinal column vitality); Seventh (Crown) Neuro-Endocrine Center (Chakra).

PC 8 (Pericardium 8, Construction Palace) — At the center of the palm between the 2nd and 3rd metacarpal bones, located by bending the third finger to touch the palm.

Huato Jiaji – about one finger width lateral to the depressions below the spinous processes of the 12 thoracic, 5 lumbar, and 7 cervical vertebrae; these points are sounded in order to stimulate the spinal nerves which makes them quite useful for harmonizing the Autonomic Nervous System. We also extend the application along all of the jia ji (points along the spine): up the cervical spine to the base of the skull and down to and including the Ba Liao foramina of the sacrum. Named after the legendary Chinese physician, Hua Tuo (2nd century AD), these points may be used to treat many conditions related to the back, spine and nervous system.

Ba Liao – the eight holes (foramina) of the sacrum which have an association with the 8 Ancestral Channels.

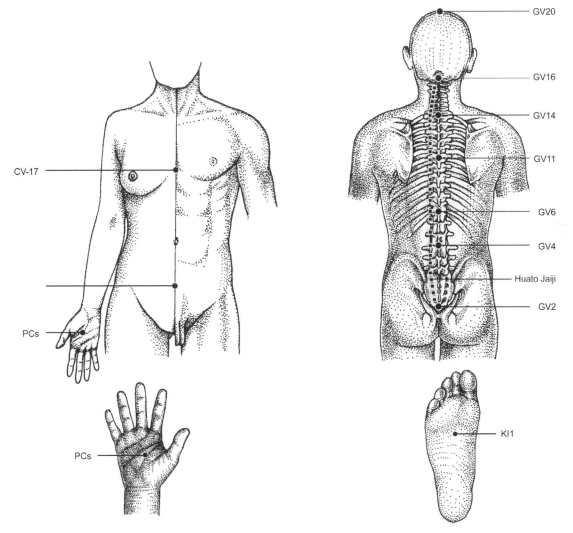

Note on Point Names:
There are multiple systems of names for the meridians, and Conception Vessel is also known as Ren, so you may see CV-4 referred to as Ren-4 in other texts. Likewise, Governor Vessel is known as Du, and GV-20 becomes Du-20. Finally Pericardium is sometimes called Heart Protector or Master of the Heart, and PC-8 becomes MH-8. In Worsley's Five Element school of Chinese medicine, the meridians have completely different names, which are not listed here.

Acupuncture Points

Acupoints are located in depressions between 1-5 square millimeters that can be found by palpation, and frequently are sensitive. Scientifically measured, they have lowered resistance and high conductivity, and consist of a vertical column of loose connective tissue which contains a large lymphatic trunk, a large arteriole, and a satellite vein. These thin-walled vessels are surrounded by netlike arrangements of nerve fibers, both myelinated and unmyelinated. A high concentration of perineural cells and micro-vesicles can be found where the sympathetic nerve endings meet the walls of the vessels. Sometimes an acupoint is called a "micro-chakra" because they are energy vortices which provide access to the flow of qi (vital energy force), and are associated with points where energy strands cross each other seven times.

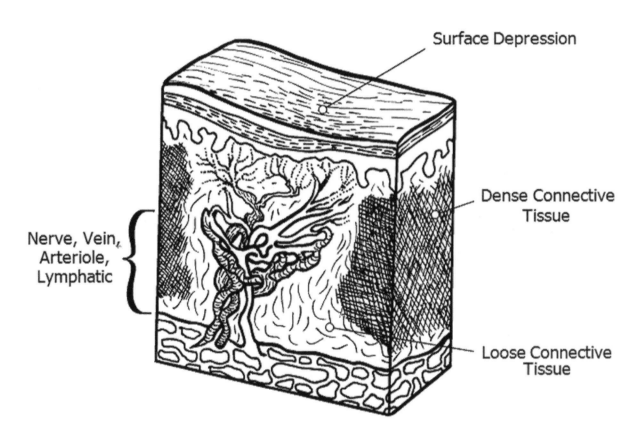

ACUPUNCTURE POINT CROSS-SECTION

Measurements: CUN

Measurements are made in "cun" or "body inches" from known body landmarks such as a bony prominence or another acupuncture point. The definition of cun is the widest distance between the ends of the interphalangeal creases on the radial surface of the client's middle finger, which is equal to the greatest width of the distal phalanx of the client's thumb. The width of the index and middle fingers at the dorsal skin crease of the proximal interphalangeal (PIP) joint of the middle finger is 1.5 cun. All four fingers held close together are 3 cun at the level of the dorsal skin crease of the PIP joint of the middle finger.

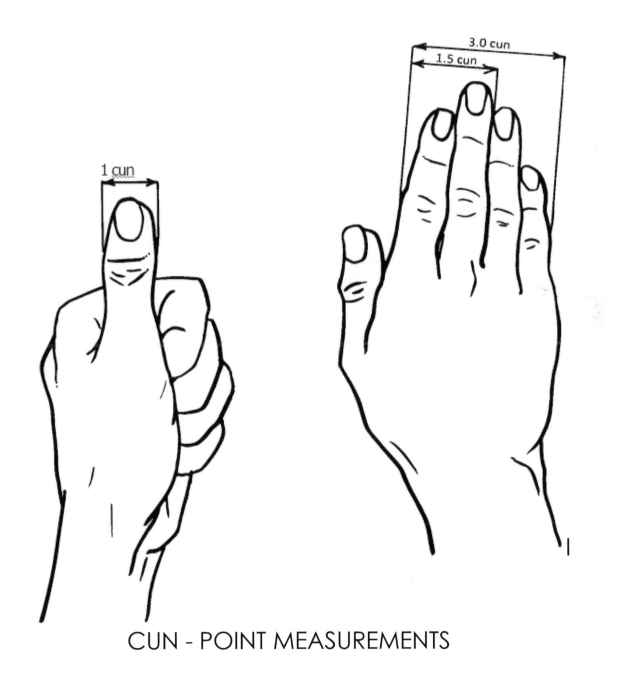

CUN - POINT MEASUREMENTS

Quick Guide - Forks & Oils

Bible Oils - 10 forks

Forks:		Essential Oils	
Low Om	High Om	Three Wise Men®	Cedarwood/Onycha
Om x 2	High Jupiter	Hyssop	Galbanum/Sandalwood
Zodiac Earth	**High Chiron Healer**	Myrtle	Cistus/Cassia
Low Chiron Healer	Angelic Om	Spikenard/Myrrh	Frankincense
Chiron Healer		Cypress	Balsam Fir

Brain - 10 forks

Forks:		Essential Oils	
Low Om	High Om 1	Valor®	Cardamom
Om x 2	High Full Sidereal Moon	Oregano	M-Grain®
Sun	High Jupiter	Thyme	Peace & Calming®
Zodiac Platonic Earth	**High Mercury**	Clarity®	Peppermint
Uranus			

Classic - 10 forks

Forks:		Essential Oils	
Low Om	High Om	Valor®	Wintergreen
Om x 2	High Full Sidereal Moon	Oregano	Marjoram
Sun	High Jupiter	Thyme	Cypress
Zodiac Platonic Earth	High Mars	Basil	Peppermint
Neptune			

Colon & Digestion - 10 forks

Forks:		Essential Oils	
Low Om	High Om	Valor®	Wintergreen
Om x 2	High Full Sidereal Moon	Oregano	Marjoram
Sun	High Jupiter	Thyme	Cypress
Zodiac Platonic Earth	**High Earth Day**	Basil	Peppermint
Pluto			

Heart/Circulation - 10 forks

Forks:

Low Om	High Om	
Ohm x 2	**High Uranus**	
Sun	**High Sign**	
Zodiac Platonic Earth	**Angelic Sun**	
Venus		

Essential Oils

Valor	Clove
Oregano	Aroma Life®
Thyme	Cypress
Goldenrod	Nutmeg

Hormone Balance/Female - 10 forks

Forks:

Low Om	High Om
Om x 2	High Jupiter
Sun	**High Saturn**
Zodiac Platonic Earth	**High Venus**
New Moon	

Essential Oils

Valor®	Fleabane
Oregano	EndoFlex®
Thyme	ClarySage
Dragon Time®	Peppermint

Hormone Balance/Male - 10 forks

Forks:

Low Om	High Om
Om x 2	High Jupiter
Sun	**High Saturn**
Zodiac Platonic Earth	**High Venus**
New Moon	

Essential Oils

Valor®	Blue Yarrow
Oregano	Mister®
Thyme	Myrtle
Lavender	Peppermint

Joints & Bones - 12 forks

Forks:

Low Om	High Om
Om x 2	High Full Sidereal Moon
Sun	High Jupiter
Zodiac Platonic Earth	High Mars
Mars	**Mercury**
Saturn	

Essential Oils

Valor®	Wintergreen
Oregano	PanAway®
Thyme	Spruce
Helichrysum	Peppermint

Liver - 10 forks

Forks:

Low Om	High Om
Om x 2	High Full Sidereal Moon
Sun	**High Pluto**
Zodiac Platonic Earth	**High Zodiac Platonic Earth**
Jupiter	

Essential Oils

Valor®	German Chamomile
Oregano	Juvaflex®
Thyme	Ledum
Carrot Seed	Peppermint

Longevity - 10 forks

Forks:

Low Om	High Om
Om x 2	High Full Sidereal Moon
Sun	High Jupiter
Zodiac Platonic Earth	**High Neptune**
Earth Day	

Essential Oils

Valor®	Clove
Oregano	Longevity®
Thyme	Frankincense
Orange	Peppermint

Lung - 10 forks

Forks:

Low Om	High Om
Om x 2	High Full Sidereal Moon
Sun	High Jupiter
Zodiac Platonic Earth	**High New Synodic Moon**
Full Sidereal Moon	

Essential Oils

Valor®	Melrose®
Oregano	Raven®
Thyme	Myrtle
Eucalyptus Radiata	Ravensara

*The tuning forks listed in plain type are from the Cassic Set, and the tuning forks listed in **bold type** are from the sets for each particular System. All of the Systems use V-6, Ortho Ease® and Aroma Siez® oils.*

Bible Oils

QUICK REFERENCE RAINDROP OUTLINE

Forks:		Essential Oils	
Low Om	High Om	Three Wise Men®	Cedarwood/Onycha
Om x 2	High Jupiter	Hyssop	Galbanum/Sandalwood
Zodiac Platonic Earth	**High Chiron Healer**	Myrtle	Cistus/Cassia
Low Chiron Healer	**Angelic Om**	Spikenard/Myrrh	Frankincense
Chiron Healer		Cypress	White Angelica

1. **Facilitator: Apply White Angelica to self on shoulders, back of neck, thymus.**
   Apply Om Unison to self at CV-4 (Origin Pass) for grounding.

2. **HAVE CLIENT LIE FACE UP. ESTABLISH ENERGY BALANCE:**
   Listen to Om Unison (2 Om forks) (hold tuning forks at least 6" from client's ears).
   THREE WISE MEN®: Rub on Shoulders (1-2 drops/shoulder) and Feet (1-2 drops/foot),
      R hand/R foot, L hand/L foot; R hand/R shoulder, L hand/L shoulder.
      Hold until you feel the energy balance left and right.
   Apply Om Unison (1 Om fork to the sole of each foot) at KI-1 (Gushing Spring).

3. **VIBRATIONAL VITA FLEX on Spinal Reflex Area of Feet (1-3 drops each oil to each foot)**
HYSSOP	MYRTLE	SPIKENARD
CYPRESS	CEDARWOOD	GALBANUM
CISTUS	FRANKINCENSE	

   Apply the Chiron Healer Major 2nd (Om and Chiron Healer forks) with Om at CV-4 (Origin Pass) on the abdomen four finger-widths below the umbilicus, and Chiron Healer at CV-17 (Chest Center) in the center of the chest level with the 4th rib. Then apply the Chiron Healer Major 2nd (Om and Chiron Healer forks) with Om at CV-17 (Chest Center) and Chiron Healer at GV-24.5 (Yin Tang) between the eyebrows.
   • HAVE CLIENT ROLL OVER TO A FACE DOWN POSITION

4. **HYSSOP:** Raindrop V-6 (6" above) 4-6 drops from sacrum to atlas.
      Raindrop (6" above) 1-2 drops Hyssop from sacrum to atlas.
      Feather stroke 3" straight up spine. Repeat with 6" then 12" strokes.
   MYRTLE: Raindrop (6" above) 1-2 drops Myrtle from sacrum to atlas.
      Feather stroke 3" straight up spine. Repeat with 6" then 12" strokes.
      Feather straight to sides in each position.
      Feather with full length strokes up and out, off the shoulders.
   Apply the Low Chiron Healer Major 2nd (Low Om and Low Chiron Healer forks) with the Low Om on GV-2 (Low Back Shu) at base of sacrum and Low Chiron Healer fork on GV-11 (Spirit Path) below T-5. Then apply Low Om on GV-11 and Low Chiron Healer on GV-20 on the crown of the head.

5. SPIKENARD(MYRRH), CYPRESS, and CEDARWOOD(ONYCHA)

Myrrh at GV-4, Raindrop/feather stroke Spikenard up spine, as in Step 4 (Hyssop).

Raindrop/feather stroke Cypress up the spine, as in Step 4 (Hyssop).

Onycha at GV-11, Raindrop/feather stroke Cedarwood up spine, as in Step 4 (Hyssop).

Finger circles (after all oils are applied).

Apply Zodiac Platonic 3rd (Om and Zodiac Platonic Earth forks) wherever muscle knots are found. Apply the Zodiac Platonic 3rd to the bank of muscles next to the spine, one side at a time. Walk up this band with the forks, moving about 2-3" each time, with Om closer to the feet and Zodiac Platonic Earth closer to the head. When completed, apply Om at the bottom of the band and Zodiac Platonic Earth at the top of the band.

6. GALBANUM(SANDALWOOD)

Sandalwood at GV-16, then raindrop 1-2 drops Galbanum (6" above) from sacrum to atlas.

Feather stroke 3" once straight up spine. Repeat with 6" then 12" strokes.

Thumb Vitaflex up spine.

Saw Maneuver up spine.

Stretch and Quiver up spine.

Apply the Chiron Healer Major 2nd (Om and Chiron Healer forks) on the Huato Jiaji points up the spine from sacrum to base of skull, alternating the Chiron Healer and Om forks on either side of the spine up to the atlas, then hold both forks at the crown of the head, GV-20.

7. ORTHO EASE®

Apply to entire back, followed by large circles with palms.

Palm Slide up & down the back. Apply more Ortho Ease® if needed.

Sound the High Jupiter 4th (High Om and High Jupiter forks) and move in a DN-8 figure over the client, from feet to crown, then back down off the feet.

8. CISTUS(CASSIA/V6)

Cassia in V6 at GV-4, then raindrop 1-2 drops Cistus (6" above) from sacrum to atlas.

Feather stroke 3" straight up spine. Repeat with 6" then 12" strokes.

Arched feather stroke 3" straight up spine. Repeat with 6" then 12" strokes.

Feather with full length strokes up and out, off the shoulders.

Sound the High Chiron Healer Major 2nd (High Om and High Chiron Healer forks) and move in a DN-8 figure over the client, from feet to crown, then down off the feet.

9. FRANKINCENSE

Raindrop (6" above) V-6 from sacrum to atlas. Add 1-3 drops Frankincense. Feather as with Cistus.

10. WARM COMPRESS

Apply hot compress; cool compress for MS clients.

Sound the High Om Octave (High Om and Angelic Om forks) in the shape of a Tetrahedron (GV-20, PC-8 and GV-11 as anchor points). Tap the forks together over the body about 24"above GV-11 (Spirit Path), then move Angelic Om to GV-20 (Hundred Convergences) while High Om stays above GV-11. Bring the forks together again above GV-11, then separate and take each fork to PC-8 (Construction Palace), one fork above each of the palms. Bring the forks together again about 24" above GV-11, take them together down to GV-20, separate them so that each fork goes to one of the palms above PC-8, and bring them together between the palms, then back up to starting position above GV-11.

Apply the Om Octave (Low Om and Om forks) to the sole of each foot at KI-1 (Gushing Spring).

11 & 12   EVALUATE AND GIVE WATER

The Bible Oils Journey
Through the New Testament

There are many ways to arrange the application of the Twelve Oils of Ancient Scripture into a VIBRATIONAL RAINDROP TECHNIQUE protocol. Of the several possible protocols that were tried, this is the arrangement which I liked best. As I studied the individual oils, their chemistry and traditional uses, a pattern began to emerge. Many of these oils have mucolytic and lung decongesting properties, a quality that would be needed as the lungs filled with water, hanging from the Cross. Some of them are hemostatic to stop the bleeding from wounds. And a few are especially noted to assist in a spiritually elevated state.

Three Wise Men

We begin the journey with the blend **Three Wise Men** as Jesus is born in a stable surrounded by farm animals. Three Wise Men has a balancing effect similar to Valor, as well as releasing emotional trauma. Jesus was visited by Magi from the east, who followed a new star to find the baby Jesus. Their gifts of Frankincense and Myrrh are in this blend; the third gift, gold, is thought to have been Fir, more precious than gold itself in that time. The facilitator of this Raindrop anoints herself with Balsam Fir to prepare for the healing. Jesus' great role of Savior is proclaimed by Simeon and Anna in the temple in Jerusalem.

Hyssop

Much of the early life of Jesus is in obscurity, until His mission begins with baptism by his cousin, John the Baptist, in the River Jordan. This is a deep cleansing with euphoric confirmations, and **hyssop** and myrtle essential oils are used in place of Oregano and Thyme. Before His ministry can truly begin, Jesus must undergo a profound test from God: He retreats into the wilderness and is tempted three times by Satan. Each temptation clarifies what it means to be the Son of God, and he emerges with knowledge of His mission and trust in God.

Myrtle

Myrtle represents great internal strength, which would be needed as Jesus is tested by Satan. Myrtle represents the masculine principle in the universe, appropriately for the Son of God. In the Old Testament, Esther (whose Hebrew name was Hadassah, meaning myrtle) showed immense internal strength as her actions saved her people from annihilation by the Persians at that time.

Cypress

Thus began Christ's ministry of many healings and miracles. **Cypress** is applied at this time because of its ability to ease emotional trauma, as well as reprogram cells to restore health with its high content of monoterpenes. Our physical illnesses always have a spiritual and emotional imbalance that needs to be healed in order for the physical to truly be well.

Spikenard

We use **spikenard** in the Bible Oils Raindrop as we move into the time of Jesus's ministry before his death, and several different occasions when he was anointed with spikenard and myrrh, on the head as well as on the feet. There are several references in the Bible which refer to separate episodes of anointing: one before the Passover in the house of Simon the Leper on His head *(Matthew 26:6-13, Mark 14:3-9)*, another in the house of Lazarus before the Passover on His feet *(John 12:3-7)*, and another early in His ministry *(Luke 7:37-49)*.

Myrrh

Myrrh is mentioned in the Bible more times than any other oil! Myrrh works well with any other oil and increases the other oils' aroma without overcoming it. It is synergistic with any oil with which it is mixed. Myrrh is the first oil to be mentioned in the Bible in the story of Joseph *(Genesis 37:25)*, as well as the last oil mentioned in the Bible *(Revelations 18:13)*. It was one of the first and last oils to be offered to Jesus: first at His birth, and last at the cross before His death. May be placed on the umbilicus and used with the Om/Chiron Major 2nd tuning forks to symbolically cut off generational "curses" inherited from ancestors.

Matthew 2:11 – "And when they were come into the house, they saw the young child with Mary his mother, and fell down, and worshipped him: and when they had opened their treasures, they presented unto him gifts; gold, and frankincense and myrrh." Gold is sometimes thought to refer to Balsam fir, which was as precious as gold in those times.

John 19:39-42 – "And there came also Nicodemus, which at the first came to Jesus by night, and brought a mixture of myrrh and aloes, about an hundred pound weight. Then took they the body of Jesus, and wound it in linen clothes with the spices, as the manner of the Jews is to bury. Now in the place where he was crucified there was a garden; and in the garden a new sepulchre, wherein was never man yet laid. There laid they Jesus therefore because of the Jews' preparation day; for the sepulchre was nigh at hand."

Jesus is offered myrrh with wine: *Mark 15:23* – "And they gave him to drink wine mingled with myrrh: but he received it not when He is brought to Golgotha to be crucified."

Cedarwood

Cedarwood is used in Bible Oils Raindrop to represent Jesus carrying his cross on the way to his crucifixion. Cedarwood from Lebanon was used for cleansing, and many houses and temples were built from it. Solomon's palace and temple was known as the "House of the Forest of Lebanon." King David refers to "the cedars of Lebanon" as "the Trees of the Lord" in *Psalms 104:16*.

Ezekiel 17:3 – "And say, Thus saith the Lord God; A great eagle with great wings, long-winged, full of feathers, which had divers colors, came unto Lebanon, and took the highest branch of the cedar." And then further in *Ezekiel 17:23:* "In the mountain of the height of Israel will I plant it: and it shall bring forth boughs, and bear fruit, and be a goodly cedar: and under it shall dwell all fowl of every wing' in the shadow of the branches thereof shall they dwell." Here is the power of cedarwood to unite the tribes and peoples of the world.

Onycha

Onycha is used with cedarwood because of its wound healing abilities as well as its assistance in making choices from the heart, the true home of our Creator.

Sandalwood

Also known as "aloes" in the Bible, **sandalwood** was one of the burial oils of Jesus. *John 19:39-42* – "And there came also Nicodemus, which at the first came to Jesus by night, and brought a mixture of myrrh and aloes, about an hundred pound weight. Then took they the body of Jesus, and wound it in linen clothes with the spices, as the manner of the Jews is to bury. Now in the place where he was crucified there was a garden; and in the garden a new sepulchre, wherein was never man yet laid. There laid they Jesus therefore because of the Jews' preparation day; for the sepulchre was nigh at hand."

Sandalwood is known as an herb of gladness in the Bible, too: *Numbers 24:6, Proverbs 7:17, Psalms 45:8,* and *Song of Solomon 4:13.*

Galbanum

When **galbanum** is added to sandalwood, its frequency of 56 is elevated (sandalwood has a frequency of 96). Mentioned by Dioscorides, ancient Roman historian, as a diuretic and pain-reliever, galbanum is used to balance extreme emotions and facilitate surrender to God's will as one pursues life's purposes. It is known as the "surrendering oil." Jesus surrenders to His crucifixion for the greater good of mankind.

Cistus

Also known as the Rose of Sharon (Rock Rose), **cistus** is mentioned in *Song of Solomon 2:1* – "I am the Rose of Sharon and the Lily of the Valleys." Some people believe that the Rose of Sharon is symbolic for Jesus Himself. As He is most perfect Himself, so too is the "rose" the most perfect of all flowers. Vibrationally, the rose has a frequency of 320 MHz, the highest frequency of all essential oils. Its fragrance is calming as well as stimulating to visions and prophecies. Cistus is also a hemostatic, and may be associated with the minimal bleeding of Christ's wounds.

Cassia

Used in conjunction with Cistus/Rose of Sharon, **cassia** catalyzes the re-awakening of the life force in the mortal body, a form of resurrection. Because of its hot nature, it should be diluted with V-6 carrier oil before being applied to the Gate of Life (Ming Men) at the lumbar spine site.

Frankincense

Frankincense has been considered the premier Holy Anointing Oil in the Mideast for thousands of years, and is thought to facilitate the connection between one and the Divine. It is related to the mythical Phoenix, which built its transformational funeral pyre out of frankincense and myrrh. It is appropriate to use sacred frankincense as the final "Resurrection" oil in the anointing sequence for Bible Oils Vibrational Raindrop Technique.

BIBLE OILS VRT: Essential Oils

Vibrational Raindrop Technique is a sequence of anointing with oils and laying on of hands that brings structural and electrical alignment to the body in a relaxing and invigorating manner through the power of essential oils. There are many versions of Vibrational Raindrop Technique, and variations in the oils that are used.

Some of the Bible Raindrop oils are high in phenolic content to ward off potentially damaging viruses and bacteria while cleansing cellular receptor sites to enhance inter- and intra- cellular communications and improve overall bodily function. Most of the Bible Raindrop oils contain a variety of sesquiterpenes to assist in deleting misinformation in the DNA, as well as monoterpenes to assist in re-programming correct information into cellular memory in order to restore and maintain physical and emotional wellness.

THREE WISE MEN®

(Contains oils of sandalwood, juniper, frankincense, myrrh and spruce in an almond oil base) opens the subconscious mind through pineal stimulation to release deep-seated and intergenerational trauma. It is high in sesquiterpenes which are able to cross the blood/brain barrier and can increase the oxygenation of the limbic system in the brain. The limbic system is the home of emotions, which can be released and enhance spiritual consciousness. Also contains large amounts of monoterpenes, which can reprogram cells back to God's original perfection. This blend has a frequency of 72 Mhz.

HYSSOP *(Hyssopus officinalis)*

Family: Lamiaceae. Is a mucolytic, decongestant, expectorant and purifier. Useful for asthma, respiratory infections, coughs and wounds. It's high in phenolic ketones to cleanse cellular receptor sites, and monoterpenes which can reprogram correct information back into cells. Its aroma stimulates creativity and meditation by its moderate amount of sesquiterpenes. Hyssop has an affinity with the Lung meridian. It clears Lung Heat such as bronchitis, and can also be used to purify the home.

Bible References:

Exodus 12:22, Leviticus 12:22, 14:4, 6, 49, 51, 52; Numbers 19:6, 18; I Kings 4:33; Hebrews 9:19.

In Psalms 51:7, King David says, "Purge me with hyssop, and I shall be clean: wash me, and I shall be whiter than snow." It is never to late for repentance and forgiveness which lead to true healing.

John 19:29 – "Now there was set a vessel full of vinegar: and they filled a sponge with vinegar, and put it upon hyssop, and put it to his mouth." Jesus was offered a sponge soaked with sour wine extended on a hyssop branch, while on the cross. Hyssop may have been able to ease the lung congestion and edema of death on the cross as well as soothe the spirit.

MYRTLE *(Myrtus communis)*

Family: Myrtaceae (myrtle); an expectorant and anti-infectious, is excellent for clearing the airways, and is used for bronchitis, coughs, tuberculosis and other pulmonary complaints. Contains 31-48% oxides, 30-45% monoterpenes.

Dry and cool, Myrtle clears Lung Heat and astringes leakage of qi and Blood such as sweating, bleeding, diarrhea and hemorrhoids. It is calming as a nervine as well as elevating and euphoric. It also represents the masculine principle in the universe, Yang energy.

Biblical references:

Nehemiah 8:15; Isaiah 41:19, 55:13; Zechariah 1:8, 10, 11.

Esther 2:7 – "And he brought up Hadassah, that is, Esther, his uncle's daughter: for she had neither father nor mother, and the maid was fair and beautiful; whom Mordecai, when her father and mother were dead, took for his own daughter." Esther was originally named Hadassah, which means myrtle, and received the name of Esther (a form of the Persian name Satarah meaning star) when she entered the royal harem of King Ahasuerus in Susa (Shoushan). It was Esther's bravery that saved the Jews of Persia from massacre.

In Jewish mysticism, the myrtle is one of four sacred plants of Sukkot, the Feast of Tabernacles, and represents those who do good deeds despite not having knowledge from the study of the Torah.

CYPRESS *(Cupressus sempervirens)*

Family: Cupressaceae (cypress family) is antimicrobial. Supportive of the circulatory and lymphatic systems, controls hemorrhages and relieves acute chest discomfort. Cypress can help ease the pain of loss while creating a feeling of security and grounding. Helps heal emotional trauma. 76% monoterpenes and 14% sesquiterpenes which may assist in restoring proper cellular programming to restore health and maintain wellness.

Slightly cooling, Cypress has an affinity for Lung, Spleen and Kidney meridians. It astringes fluid discharge that results from leakage of qi, such as urine, sweat, or diarrhea. Cypress ascends Spleen qi to upbear prolapse, hemorrhoids and varicose veins. Finally, it is very helpful to clear Lung heat and assists the Kidney to grasp Lung qi in wheezing and bedwetting.

Biblical references:

Isaiah 44:14 – " He heweth him down cedars, and taketh the cypress and the oak, which he strengtheneth for himself among the trees of the forest: he planteth an ash, and the rain doth nourish it."

SPIKENARD *(Nardostachys jatamansi)*

Family: Valerianaceae; purifying and cleansing, spikenard is also relaxing and soothing, and can regenerate the skin. Contains 36-50% sesquiterpenes, 37-45% monoterpenes, and 6-11% sesquiterpenols.

Spikenard is cooling with an affinity for Liver and Pericardium meridians. It clears Heart fire (palpitations, tachycardia, arrhythmias, agitation) and subdues Liver wind (headaches, seizures). Apply to CV 4 below the umbilicus or to CV 17 on the chest for soothing and calming the Shen.

Biblical references:

Song of Solomon 1:12, 4:13, 4:14. Spikenard was one of the most precious oils in ancient times for kings, priests and high initiates.

Matthew 26:6-13, Mark 14:3-9, John 12:3-7, and Luke 7:37-49, John 12:3, Luke 7:37-49.

MYRRH *(Commiphora myrrha)*

Family: Burseraceae; is a powerful antioxidant, antitumoral, anti-inflammatory used for healing of skin wounds. Its fragrance promotes spiritual awareness, is uplifting, and contains 62% sesquiterpenes that stimulate the limbic system of the brain, as well as the hypothalamus, pineal and pituitary glands. Myrrh vibrates to a high frequency of 105 Mhz.

Cooling in nature, myrrh has an affinity for the Lung, Spleen and Stomach meridians. It clears Lung and Stomach heat symptoms such as difficult cough, wheezing, and copious sputum, invigorates the blood for bruises, and promotes healing of wounds.

Biblical references:

Genesis 37:25, 43:11; Exodus 30:23; Esther 2:12; Psalms 45:8; Proverbs 7:17; Son of Solomon 1:13, 3:6, 4:6, 4:14, 5:1, 5:5, 5:13.
Matthew 2:11, John 19:39-42, Mark 15:23.

CEDARWOOD *(Cedrus atlantica)*

Family: Pinaceae; has the highest amount of sesquiterpenes of any oil (98%) to cross the blood-brain barrier to deprogram misinformation and increase oxygen at cellular levels. Enhances deep sleep by stimulating melatonin, promotes mental clarity. It is used for bronchitis, tuberculosis, and hair loss. We use this oil in Bible Oils Raindrop to represent Jesus carrying his cross on the way to his crucifixion.

Leviticus 14:4, 6, 49, 51, 52; Numbers 19:6, Ezekiel 17:3, Ezekiel 17:23.

In ancient times, cedarwood was used for ritual cleaning after touching anything "unclean" such as a dead body or something considered to have evil spirits. Mentioned in Leviticus in conjunction with hyssop to be used for cleansing of leprosy by applying to the tip of the right ear, right thumb and right toe. May be the most ancient of distilled oils, and was used for embalming more than 5000 years ago.

There are many, many references to cedarwood as the material out of which houses and temples are made (Samuel, I Kings, Chronicles, Ezekiel, and more), of which Solomon's palace and temple was known as the "House of the Forest of Lebanon." King David refers to "the cedars of Lebanon" as "the Trees of the Lord" in Psalms 104:16.

ONYCHA *(Styrax benzoin)*

Family: Styracaceae; rich in esters and aldehydes which give it a pleasant vanilla-like smell, it is used for bronchitis, colds, coughs as well for skin wounds. Onycha helps one to make choices from the heart, and holds our energies in resonance with the Source fire. This is one of Moses' anointing oils, along with galbanum and stacte.

Biblical references:

Exodus 30:34 – "And the Lord said unto Moses, Take unto thee sweet spices, stacte, and onycha, and galbanum; these sweet spices with pure frankincense of each shall there be a like weight."

GALBANUM *(Ferula gummosa)*

Family: Apiaceae; esteemed for its medicinal and spiritual properties, galbanum supports the kidneys, lungs and nervous system. Because of its harmonic balancing nature, it may assist with spiritual awareness. Especially rich in monoterpenes (50-95%) to reprogram cells back to God's original perfection. It's frequency of 56 can be elevated when combined with frankincense or sandalwood (frequency 96). Mentioned by Dioscorides, ancient Roman historian, as a diuretic and pain-reliever. Galbanum is used to balance extreme emotions and facilitate surrender to God's will as one pursues life's purpose. It is known as the "surrendering oil."

Biblical references:

Exodus 30:34 – "And the Lord said unto Moses, Take unto thee sweet spices, stacte, and onycha, and galbanum; these sweet spices with pure frankincense of each shall there be a like weight."

Cooling by nature, Galbanum has an affinity with the Liver and Spleen meridians. It regulates Liver qi and expels damp-phlegm and damp bi-obstruction at the extremities, as well as supports and strengthens Lung qi. It can promote cell regeneration.

SANDALWOOD *(Santalum album)*

Family: Santalaceae, has been used for over 4,000 years in Ayurvedic medicine, Buddhism and Islam for meditation and spiritual growth. Like the tree itself, the oil inspires one to be able to extract nourishment and survive in adverse circumstances; and its concentration is richest and most abundant in its heartwood, the deepest part of the tree. It enhances deep sleep through the release of melatonin and may help remove negative programming from the cells. It contains the fourth highest concentration of sesquiterpenes (90%) of all the oils which cross the blood-brain barrier.

Also known as "aloes" in the Bible, sandalwood was one of the burial oils of Jesus. In Ayurvedic literature, sandalwood is considered to have a sympathetic resonance with "All That Is." As the Indian poet Rabindranath Tagore says, "The Sandal Tree as if to prove, How sweet to conquer Hate, love, Perfumes the axe that lays it low." ("Sacred Sandalwood" by Christopher McMahon).

Biblical references:

John 19:39-42 – "And there came also Nicodemus, which at the first came to Jesus by night, and brought a mixture of myrrh and aloes, about an hundred pound weight. Then took they the body of Jesus, and wound it in linen clothes with the spices, as the manner of the Jews is to bury. Now in the place where he was crucified there was a garden; and in the garden a new sepulchre, wherein was never man yet laid. There laid they Jesus therefore because of the Jews' preparation day; for the sepulchre was nigh at hand."

Some other references which refer to Sandalwood/aloes as an herb of gladness include Numbers 24:6, Proverbs 7:17, Psalms 45:8, and Song of Solomon 4:13.

Sandalwood is slightly cooling with an affinity for the Lung, Spleen, Kidney and Bladder meridians. It calms the Shen/spirit (apply directly to CV 17) and opens the diaphragm (apply to CV 12) to move qi such as with a cough or to expel phlegm.

CISTUS *(Cistus ladanifer)*

Family: Cistaceae is antiseptic, immune enhancing because of its phenols, supportive of body's natural defenses. High in monoterpenes to assist in reprogramming correct information into cells, and has been studied for its effects on cellular regeneration. Its fragrance is calming as well as stimulating to visions and prophecies.

With an affinity for Lung, Spleen and Kidney meridians, cistus is a hemostatic and can stop bleeding. It can regulate the Liver when overacting on the Spleen meridians, such as with hemorrhoids or menstrual problems. It also can Expel Cold on the surface (by astringing the Yang) such as with nasal congestion.

Biblical references:

Also known as the Rose of Sharon (Rock Rose) mentioned in Song of Solomon 2:1 – "I am the Rose of Sharon and the Lily of the Valleys." Some people believe that the Rose of Sharon is symbolic for Jesus himself. As He is most perfect Himself, so too is the "rose" the most perfect of all flowers. Vibrationally, the rose has a frequency of 320 MHz, the highest frequency of all essential oils.

CASSIA *(Cinnamomun cassia)*

Family: Lauraceae can be high in aldehydes and phenols, which can cleanse receptor sites. Because of its hot nature, it should be diluted with V-6 carrier oil before being applied to Ming Men at the lumbar spine site. Used in conjunction with Cistus/Rose of Sharon, it catalyzes the re-awakening of the life force in the mortal body, a form of resurrection.

Cassia is hot by nature with an affinity to the Liver, Spleen, Kidney and Bladder meridians. It can warm the Middle and Lower Heater to expel Cold and tonify Yang; it can strengthen the Ming-Men Fire.

FRANKINCENSE *(Boswellia carteri)*

Family: Burseraceae (frankincense); antitumoral, immunostimulant, antidepressant; increases spiritual awareness, promotes meditation, improves attitude. Contains 64-90% monoterpenes, 5-10% sesquiterpenes, which stimulate the limbic system of the brain (the center of memory and emotions), and the hypothalamus, pineal and pituitary glands. Particularly useful for asthma and ulcers, and may also be used for many types of inflammatory conditions. This is one of the most important oils for anointing.

Slightly cooling and drying, Frankincense has an affinity for the Lung, Heart and Kidney meridians. Use it for Lung Heat with Chest Qi Stasis symptoms of agitation, anxiety and irritability. Clears heat in the Lungs with coughing or wheezing, Stomach with ulcers, and Kidneys with cystitis. It can also reduce swelling and treat non-healing wounds, ulcers and scars. The ability of frankincense to the Divine Spirit is related to its Yin organ, the Lung, which opens upward and outward to God. It is through the first breath that we are born, and with the last breath that we depart this physical realm.

Biblical references:

There are over 52 references to frankincense in the Bible! Also known as "olibanum" or oil from Lebanon, frankincense is derived from the words for "real incense" in Medieval French. Frankincense has been considered the premier Holy Anointing Oil in the Middle East for thousands of years, and is thought to facilitate the connection between one and the Divine. It is related to the mythical Phoenix, which built its transformational funeral pyre out of frankincense and myrrh.

It was one of the sacred and precious gifts given to Jesus at His birth.

Matthew 2:11 — "And when they were come into the house, they saw the young child with Mary his mother, and fell down, and worshipped him: and when they had opened their treasures, they presented unto him gifts; gold, and frankincense and myrrh." Gold is sometimes thought to refer to Balsam fir, which was as precious as gold in those times.

ORTHO EASE®

(a massage base oil of wheat germ, grape seed, almond, olive, and vitamin E containing essential oils of wintergreen, juniper, marjoram, red thyme, vetiver, peppermint, eucalyptus, and lemongrass) is used in European hospitals, formulated to soothe muscle aches and minor swelling. Contains natural antioxidants.

BIBLE OILS VRT: Forks & Intervals

The tuning forks of the Bible Oils Vibrational Raindrop Technique focus on the intervals created with the use of the Chiron tuning forks combined with Om, to create a Major 2nd Interval.

Unison, 1:1

Om/Om – centering, rooting and grounding. We begin the Raindrop journey from a firm, grounded place within.

Major 2nd, 8:9

Om/Chiron Healer or High Om/High Chiron Healer or Low Om/Low Chiron Healer – dense but warmer than the Minor Second; allows access to deep wounds and scars of a physical, emotional, or spiritual nature to transform and repair. Occurs between consonant intervals (octave, 5th, 4th and 3rd) and dissonant intervals (2nd), and thus is the space between harmony and disharmony.

Octave, 1:2

Om/Low Om or High Om/Angelic Om – Perfect Octave, dreams come true; brings feelings of comfort, completeness, and creates a sense of unity with All That Is. Thus ends our journey of healing with a Vibrational Raindrop Technique session.

BRAIN: Vibrational Raindrop Technique

QUICK REFERENCE RAINDROP OUTLINE

Forks:		Essential Oils	
Low Om	High Om	Valor®	Cardamom
Om x 2	High Full Sidereal Moon	Oregano	M-Grain®
Sun	High Jupiter	Thyme	Peace & Calming®
Zodiac Platonic Earth	**High Mercury**	Clarity®	Peppermint
Uranus		White Angelica	

1. **Facilitator: Apply White Angelica to self on shoulders, back of neck, thymus.**
   Apply Om Unison to self at CV-4 (Origin Pass) for grounding.

2. **HAVE CLIENT LIE FACE UP. ESTABLISH ENERGY BALANCE:**
   Listen to Om Unison (2 Om forks) (hold tuning forks at least 6" from client's ears).
   <u>VALOR®:</u> Rub on Shoulders (1-2 drops/shoulder) and Feet (1-2 drops/foot),
      R hand/R foot, L hand/L foot; R hand/R shoulder, L hand/L shoulder.
      Hold until you feel the energy balance left and right.
   Apply Om Unison (1 Om fork to the sole of each foot) at KI-1 (Gushing Spring).

3. **VIBRATIONAL VITA FLEX on Spinal Reflex Area of Feet** (1-3 drops each oil to each foot)
VALOR®	OREGANO	THYME CLARITY®
CARDAMOM	M-GRAIN®	
PEACE & CALMING®	PEPPERMINT	

   Apply the Om Octave (Om and Low Om forks) with Low Om at CV-4 (Origin Pass) on the abdomen four finger-widths below the umbilicus, and Om at CV-17 (Chest Center) in the center of the chest level with the 4th rib. Then apply the Om Octave (Om and Low Om forks) with Low Om at CV-17 (Chest Center) and Om at GV-24.5 (Yin Tang) between the eyebrows.
   - **HAVE CLIENT ROLL OVER TO A FACE DOWN POSITION**

4. **OREGANO:** Raindrop V-6 (6" above) 4-6 drops from sacrum to atlas.
      Raindrop (6" above) 1-2 drops Oregano from sacrum to atlas.
      Feather stroke 3" straight up spine. Repeat with 6" then 12" strokes.
   THYME: Raindrop (6" above) 1-2 drops Thyme from sacrum to atlas.
      Feather stroke 3" straight up spine. Repeat with 6" then 12" strokes.
      Feather straight to sides in each position.
      Feather with full length strokes up and out, off the shoulders.
   Apply the Solar 7th (Low Om and Sun forks) with the Low Om on GV-2 (Low Back Shu) at base of sacrum and Sun fork on GV-11 (Spirit Path) below T-5. Then apply Low Om on GV-11 and Sun on GV-20 on the crown of the head.

5. CLARITY®, CARDAMOM, and M-GRAIN®

Raindrop and feather each oil on spine, as in Step 4 (Oregano).

Finger circles (after all three oils are applied).

Apply Zodiac Platonic 3rd (Om and Zodiac Platonic Earth forks) wherever muscle knots are found. Apply the Zodiac Platonic 3rd to the bank of muscles next to the spine, one side at a time. Walk up this band with the forks, moving about 2-3" each time, with Om closer to the feet and Zodiac Platonic Earth closer to the head. When completed, apply Om at the bottom of the band and Zodiac Platonic Earth at the top of the band.

6. PEACE & CALMING®

Sprinkle (6" above) from sacrum to atlas.

Feather stroke 3" straight up spine. Repeat with 6" then 12" strokes.

Thumb Vitaflex up spine.

Saw Maneuver up spine.

Stretch and Quiver up spine.

Apply the Uranus 5th (Om and Uranus forks) on the Huato Jiaji points up the spine from sacrum to base of skull, alternating the Uranus and Om forks on either side of the spine up to the atlas, then hold both forks at the crown of the head, GV-20.

7. ORTHO EASE®

Apply to entire back, followed by large circles with palms.

Palm Slide up & down the back. Apply more Ortho Ease® if needed.

Sound the High Jupiter 4th (High Om and High Jupiter forks) and move in a DN-8 figure over the client, from feet to crown, then back down off the feet.

8. VALOR®

Sprinkle (6" above) from sacrum to atlas.

Feather stroke 3" straight up spine. Repeat with 6" then 12" strokes.

Arched feather stroke 3" straight up spine. Repeat with 6" then 12" strokes.

Feather with full length strokes up and out, off the shoulders.

Sound the High Mercury microtone (High Om and High Mercury forks) and move in a DN-8 figure over the client, from feet to crown, then down off the feet.

9. PEPPERMINT (Use sparingly: 1-2 drops)

Raindrop (6" above) 1-2 drops from sacrum to atlas. Feather as with Valor.

10. WARM COMPRESS

Apply hot compress; cool compress for MS clients.

Sound the High Full Sidereal Moon Major 6th (High Om and High Full Sidereal Moon forks), move in a DN-8 figure over the client from feet to crown, then down off the feet.

Apply the Om Octave (Om and Low Om forks) to the sole of each foot at KI-1 (Gushing Spring).

11 & 12   EVALUATE AND GIVE WATER.

BRAIN VRT: Essential Oils

All of the Systems-specific Vibrational Raindrop Technique protocol use Valor, oregano and thyme as the core three oils to open and close Vibrational Raindrop Technique (EDOR, 4th Ed, page 299). Basil, marjoram, wintergreen, cypress and peppermint are replaced with oils more specific to the body system being treated. Details about the specific oils used to focus on the Brain system are included below.

CLARITY®

(Contains oils of cardamom, rosemary CT cineol, peppermint, basil, bergamot, geranium, jasmine, lemon, palmarosa, Roman chamomile, rosewood and ylang ylang); promotes a clear mind and amplifies mental alertness, increases energy when tired, and brings the spirit and mind back into focus. Contains esters, oxides, transphenol (cardamom).

CARDAMOM *(Elettaria cardamomum)*

Family: Zingiberaceae; antispasmodic (neuromuscular), has been used for senility, memory problems, headaches. Supports the respiratory system, good for sinus and lung infections (contains over 32% 1,8 cineole). Steam distilled from seeds which were called "Grains of Paradise" since the Middle Ages, highly prized spice in Ancient Greece and Rome. Uplifting, energizing, refreshing. High in esters (over 50%) as well as oxides (1,8 cineole). Contains high levels of transphenol, which may generate headaches in the presence of petrochemicals or heavy metals.

Warming Cardamom has an affinity for the Lung and Spleen meridians. It harmonizes Spleen and Stomach to treat digestion problems, and transforms Dampness in Summer Heat. Especially good for Rebellious Qi and Turbid Dampness with dizziness, abdominal fullness and poor concentration.

M-GRAIN®

(Contains marjoram, lavender, peppermint, basil, Roman chamomile, and helichrysum); has been used to relieve pain from muscular headaches as well as migraine headaches; anti-inflammatory and antispasmodic. Contains monoterpenes, phenolics, sesquiterpenes.

PEACE & CALMING®

(Contains blue tansy, patchouli, tangerine, orange, and ylang ylang); promotes relaxation and a deep sense of emotional well being; helps to dampen tensions and uplift spirits. Citrus fragrances have been shown to lessen depression and increase a deep sense of security (Mie University, 1995). Contains ketones, sesquiterpenes in patchouli which stimulate the limbic center of the brain, esters and aldehydes in tangerine that are sedating and calming, monoterpenes in orange to reprogram the cells back to original perfection, and sesquiterpenes and esters in ylang ylang.

PEPPERMINT *(Mentha piperita)*

CT menthol – Family: Lamiaceae supports digestive system, respiratory system, and nervous system. Has been used for headaches. Research has shown that inhaling peppermint improves concentration and mental retention. Detoxing to the liver. A synergistic oil that supports and improves the beneficial actions of other oils used in conjunction. High in phenolics, but contains 9% sesquiterpenes. Peppermint has an affinity for the Lung and Liver meridians with its cooling energy. Clears Wind Heat of headaches, fever, sore throat, and dry cough, as well as regulates Liver qi to promote menstruation, and decongest the Liver/PMS. It also promotes the movement of Wei qi.

A Note About Sesquiterpenes:

Sesquiterpenes, a type of terpene commonly found in essential oils, are able to pass through the blood-brain barrier to enter the brain. This barrier separates our circulating blood from the brain in order to protect the brain from exposure to toxins that the rest of the body can tolerate. However, there are certain diseases that can be treated only by access via the blood-brain barrier: Alzheimer's disease, multiple sclerosis, Parkinson's disease to name a few. Sesquiterpenes are able to carry oxygen into the cells all over the body, including the brain. Both frankincense and sandalwood have significant levels of sesquiterpenes and sesquiterpenols, which can increase the oxygenation of the limbic system in the brain. This affects the pituitary and pineal glands, critical to our bodies' functioning.

It also affects the amygdala, a key player in the storage and releasing of emotional trauma. Other oils with high levels of sesquiterpenes include vetiver, vitex, cedarwood, black pepper, ylang ylang, melissa, myrrh, goldenrod, German chamomile, patchouli, ginger, spikenard, and copaiba.

BRAIN VRT: Tuning Fork Intervals

Microtone

High Om/High Mercury – creates a great deal of movement and dissonance; volatile, going between the cracks, mental illumination and communication. Mercury has an affinity with the nervous system and communication of all kinds. It also balances the sympathetic nervous system and thyroid.

Fifth, 2:3

Om/Uranus – the Electrical Fifth; opens with the electrical charge of transformation, can shatter pre¬existing conceptions and embodies the energy of freedom and independence. Mentally transformative, illuminating, inventive and break-through ideas. Uranus governs the electrical activity of the nervous system, and can calm and balance it.

CLASSIC Vibrational Raindrop Technique

QUICK REFERENCE RAINDROP OUTLINE

Forks:		Essential Oils	
Low Om	High Om	Valor®	Wintergreen
Om x 2	High Full Sidereal Moon	Oregano	Marjoram
Sun	High Jupiter	Thyme	Cypress
Zodiac Platonic Earth	High Mars	Basil	Peppermint
Neptune		White Angelica	

1. **Facilitator: Apply White Angelica to self on shoulders, back of neck, thymus.**
   Apply Om Unison to self at CV-4 (Origin Pass) for grounding.

2. **HAVE CLIENT LIE FACE UP. ESTABLISH ENERGY BALANCE:**
   Listen to Om Unison (2 Om forks) (hold tuning forks at least 6" from client's ears).
   <u>VALOR®</u>: Rub on Shoulders (1-2 drops/shoulder) and Feet (1-2 drops/foot),
       R hand/R foot, L hand/L foot; R hand/R shoulder, L hand/L shoulder.
       Hold until you feel the energy balance left and right.
   Apply Om Unison (1 Om fork to the sole of each foot) at KI-1 (Gushing Spring).

3. **VIBRATIONAL VITA FLEX on Spinal Reflex Area of Feet** (1-3 drops each oil to each foot)

OREGANO	THYME	BASIL
CYPRESS	WINTERGREEN	MARJORAM
PEPPERMINT		

   Apply the Om Octave (Om and Low Om forks) with Low Om at CV-4 (Origin Pass) on the abdomen four finger-widths below the umbilicus, and Om at CV-17 (Chest Center) in the center of the chest level with the 4th rib. Then apply the Om Octave (Om and Low Om forks) with Low Om at CV-17 (Chest Center) and Om at GV-24.5 (Yin Tang) between the eyebrows.
   - **HAVE CLIENT ROLL OVER TO A FACE DOWN POSITION**

4. **OREGANO:** Raindrop V-6 (6" above) 4-6 drops from sacrum to atlas.
       Raindrop (6" above) 1-2 drops Oregano from sacrum to atlas.
       Feather stroke 3" straight up spine. Repeat with 6" then 12" strokes.
   THYME: Raindrop (6" above) 1-2 drops Thyme from sacrum to atlas.
       Feather stroke 3" straight up spine. Repeat with 6" then 12" strokes.
       Feather straight to sides in each position.
       Feather with full length strokes up and out, off the shoulders.
   Apply the Solar 7th (Low Om and Sun forks) with the Low Om on GV-2 (Low Back Shu) at base of sacrum and Sun fork on GV-11 (Spirit Path) below T-5. Then apply Low Om on GV-11 and Sun on GV-20 on the crown of the head.

5. BASIL, WINTERGREEN, and MARJORAM

Raindrop and feather each oil on spine, as in Step 4 (Oregano).

Finger circles (after all three oils are applied).

Apply Zodiac Platonic 3rd (Om and Zodiac Platonic Earth forks) wherever muscle knots are found. Apply the Zodiac Platonic 3rd to the bank of muscles next to the spine, one side at a time. Walk up this band with the forks, moving about 2-3" each time, with Om closer to the feet and Zodiac Platonic Earth closer to the head. When completed, apply Om at the bottom of the band and Zodiac Platonic Earth at the top of the band.

6. CYPRESS

Sprinkle (6" above) from sacrum to atlas.

Feather stroke 3" straight up spine. Repeat with 6" then 12" strokes.

Thumb Vitaflex up spine.

Saw Maneuver up spine.

Stretch and Quiver up spine.

Apply the Neptune 5th (Om and Neptune forks) on the Huato Jiaji points up the spine from sacrum to base of skull, alternating the Neptune and Om forks on either side of the spine up to the atlas, then hold both forks at the crown of the head, GV-20.

7. ORTHO EASE®

Apply to entire back, followed by large circles with palms.

Palm Slide up & down the back. Apply more Ortho Ease® if needed.

Sound the High Jupiter 4th (High Om and High Jupiter forks) and move in a DN-8 figure over the client, from feet to crown, then back down off the feet.

8. VALOR®

Sprinkle (6" above) from sacrum to atlas.

Feather stroke 3" straight up spine. Repeat with 6" then 12" strokes.

Arched feather stroke 3" straight up spine. Repeat with 6" then 12" strokes.

Feather with full length strokes up and out, off the shoulders.

Sound the High Mars minor 2nd (High Om and High Mars forks) and move in a DN-8 figure over the client, from feet to crown, then down off the feet.

9. PEPPERMINT (Use sparingly: 1-2 drops)

Raindrop (6" above) 1-2 drops from sacrum to atlas. Feather as with Valor.

10. WARM COMPRESS

Apply hot compress; cool compress for MS clients.

Sound the High Full Sidereal Moon Major 6th (High Om and High Full Sidereal Moon forks), move in a DN-8 figure over the client from feet to crown, then down off the feet.

Apply the Om Octave (Om and Low Om forks) to the sole of each foot at KI-1 (Gushing Spring).

11 & 12   EVALUATE AND GIVE WATER.

CLASSIC VRT:
A Rainbow of Forks & Intervals

The ten tuning forks included in the Classic Vibrational Raindrop Technique are specifically chosen to allow a full spectrum of musical intervals to be toned.

Unison, 1:1

Om/Om – centering, rooting, and grounding. We begin from a firm, grounded place within.

Minor 2nd, 15:16

High Om/High Mars – harsh; carrier of considerable energetic potential, propels the mind, body and spirit into action with power and initiative to remove obstacles. This interval is used near the end of the journey, when we need to mobilize our energies and courage to move and release the unnecessary burdens that we carry.

Major 3rd, 4:5

Om/Zodiac Platonic Earth – optimistic, happy; meditative, dispersive or dispelling effect, relieves mental stress, but is especially useful to relieve physical stress. This interval is used after the Trio of oils in the middle of the Raindrop session, and it is well-suited to release muscle spasms in the back, especially with Aroma Siez.

Perfect 4th, 3:4

High Om/High Jupiter – Perfect Fourth; pure, like church bells; stimulates growth, abundance and expansion. The major energetic work has been done, and we relax for a few minutes to enjoy the bounty of it all.

Perfect 5th, 2:3

Om/Neptune – a near Perfect Fifth, aptly called the Ecstatic Fifth, opens and moves the visionary to transcendental, fulfills the yearning for connection with the Infinite. Alternating these forks up the spine is the perfect energetic treatment for problems of the back, such as scoliosis or chronic pain.

Major 6th, 3:5

High Om/High Full Sidereal Moon – optimistic, less emotional than the Major 3rd; builds energy, brings a feeling of fullness and purification; the ultimate expression of Yin. Can bring a sense of magic and fulfillment, with a pull towards healing that allows one's potential to manifest. This interval is used as Peppermint pushes the oils ever deeper into healing levels. Relax and know that the cleansing and release are perfect.

Minor 7th, 5:9

Low Om/Sun – full of tensions initiative, empowerment, vitalizing and warm, unconditional love; the ultimate expression of Yang. This interval assists the core Duo of Oregano and Thyme to "heat up" the cells and cleanse them for deletion of old, redundant and useless information. These two points achieve "cranial-sacral stillpoint" from which changes can occur and a new order can be achieved.

Octave, 1:2

Low Om/Om – Perfect Octave, dreams come true; brings feelings of comfort, grounding and unity.

COLON AND DIGESTION
Vibrational Raindrop Technique

QUICK REFERENCE RAINDROP OUTLINE

Forks:		Essential Oils	
Low Om	High Om	Valor®	Tarragon
Om x2	High Full Sidereal Moon	Oregano	Di-Gize®
Sun	High Jupiter	Thyme	Fennel
Zodiac Platonic Earth	**High Earth Day**	Cumin	Spearmint
Pluto		White Angelica	

1. **Facilitator: Apply White Angelica to self on shoulders, back of neck, thymus.**
   Apply Om Unison to self at CV-4 (Origin Pass) for grounding.

2. **HAVE CLIENT LIE FACE UP. ESTABLISH ENERGY BALANCE:**
   Listen to Om Unison (2 Om forks) (hold tuning forks at least 6" from client's ears).
   <u>VALOR®</u>: Rub on Shoulders (1-2 drops/shoulder) and Feet (1-2 drops/foot),
   R hand/R foot, L hand/L foot; R hand/R shoulder, L hand/L shoulder.
   Hold until you feel the energy balance left and right.
   Apply Om Unison (1 Om fork to the sole of each foot) at KI-1 (Gushing Spring).

3. **VIBRATIONAL VITA FLEX on Spinal Reflex Area of Feet** (1-3 drops each oil to each foot)

VALOR®	OREGANO	THYME
CUMIN	TARRAGON	DI-GIZE®
FENNEL	SPEARMINT	

   Apply the Om Octave (Om and Low Om forks) with Low Om at CV-4 (Origin Pass) on the abdomen four finger-widths below the umbilicus, and Om at CV-17 (Chest Center) in the center of the chest level with the 4th rib. Then apply the Om Octave (Om and Low Om forks) with Low Om at CV-17 (Chest Center) and Om at GV-24.5 (Yin Tang) between the eyebrows.
   • **HAVE CLIENT ROLL OVER TO A FACE DOWN POSITION**

4. **OREGANO:** Raindrop V-6 (6" above) 4-6 drops from sacrum to atlas.
   Raindrop (6" above) 1-2 drops Oregano from sacrum to atlas.
   Feather stroke 3" straight up spine. Repeat with 6" then 12" strokes.
   THYME: Raindrop (6" above) 1-2 drops Thyme from sacrum to atlas.
   Feather stroke 3" straight up spine. Repeat with 6" then 12" strokes.
   Feather straight to sides in each position.
   Feather with full length strokes up and out, off the shoulders.
   Apply the Solar 7th (Low Om and Sun forks) with the Low Om on GV-2 (Low Back Shu) at base of sacrum and Sun fork on GV-11 (Spirit Path) below T-5. Then apply Low Om on GV-11 and Sun on GV-20 on the crown of the head.

5. CUMIN, TARRAGON, and DI-GIZE®

Raindrop and feather each oil on spine, as in Step 4 (Oregano).

Finger circles (after all three oils are applied).

Apply Zodiac Platonic 3rd (Om and Zodiac Platonic Earth forks) wherever muscle knots are found. Apply the Zodiac Platonic 3rd to the bank of muscles next to the spine, one side at a time. Walk up this band with the forks, moving about 2-3" each time, with Om closer to the feet and Zodiac Platonic Earth closer to the head. When completed, apply Om at the bottom of the band and Zodiac Platonic Earth at the top of the band.

6. FENNEL

Sprinkle (6" above) from sacrum to atlas.

Feather stroke 3" straight up spine. Repeat with 6" then 12" strokes.

Thumb Vitaflex up spine.

Saw Maneuver up spine.

Stretch and Quiver up spine.

Apply the Pluto microtone (Om and Pluto forks) on the Huato Jiaji points up the spine from sacrum to base of skull, alternating the Pluto and Om forks on either side of the spine up to the atlas, then hold both forks at the crown of the head, GV-20.

7. ORTHO EASE®

Apply to entire back, followed by large circles with palms.

Palm Slide up & down the back. Apply more Ortho Ease® if needed.

Sound the High Jupiter 4th (High Om and High Jupiter forks) and move in a DN-8 figure over the client, from feet to crown, then back down off the feet.

8. VALOR®

Sprinkle (6" above) from sacrum to atlas.

Feather stroke 3" straight up spine. Repeat with 6" then 12" strokes.

Arched feather stroke 3" straight up spine. Repeat with 6" then 12" strokes.

Feather with full length strokes up and out, off the shoulders.

Sound the High Earth Day Augmented 4th (High Om and High Earth Day forks) and move in a DN-8 figure over the client, from feet to crown, then down off the feet.

9. SPEARMINT

Raindrop (6" above) 1-2 drops from sacrum to atlas. Feather as with Valor.

10. WARM COMPRESS

Apply hot compress; cool compress for MS clients.

Sound the High Full Sidereal Moon Major 6th (High Om and High Full Sidereal Moon forks), move in a DN-8 figure over the client from feet to crown, then down off the feet.

Apply the Om Octave (Om and Low Om forks) to the sole of each foot at KI-1 (Gushing Spring).

11 & 12   EVALUATE AND GIVE WATER

COLON AND DIGESTION VRT:
Essential Oils

All of the Systems-specific Vibrational Raindrop Technique protocol use Valor, oregano and thyme as the core three oils to open and close Vibrational Raindrop Technique (EDOR, 4th Ed, page 299). Basil, marjoram, wintergreen, cypress and peppermint are replaced with oils more specific to the body system being treated. Details about the specific oils used to focus on the Colon/Digestion system are included below.

DI-GIZE®
(Contains tarragon, ginger, peppermint, juniper, fennel, lemongrass, anise, and patchouli); relieves digestive problems including indigestion, heartburn, gas, and bloating. Combats candida and parasite infestation.

TARRAGON *(Artemisia dracunculus)*
Family: Asteraceae; antispasmodic, antiinflammatory, antifermentation, antiparasitic, digestive aid. Used in intestinal disorders, colitis, nausea; may balance the autonomic nervous system. High in phenolic ethers (estragole) and monoterpenes.

Tarragon is warming by nature with an affinity for the Liver and Spleen meridians. It regulates Stomach qi for problems such as vomiting, hiccups, belching, flatulence, dyspepsia, and poor appetite. It can also be used for the Liver Qi Stagnation of PMS to promote menstruation.

CUMIN *(Cuminum cyminum)*
Family: Apiaceae; distilled from seeds, used for digestion and infections. Immune stimulant, liver protectant. High in monoterpenes and aldehydes.

Cumin is slightly warming with an affinity for the Liver, Spleen, and Heart meridians. It is indicated for Deficient Spleen qi symptoms of poor digestion, loose stools, abdominal distention, obesity, and edema. It can also be used to Invigorate the Blood with Deficient Heart qi symptoms of fatigue, palpitations, and low blood pressure.

FENNEL *(Foeniculum vulgare)*
Family: Apiaceae; may be used for indigestion, constipation, PMS, and balancing hormones. It may break up fluids and toxins to cleanse the tissues. High in phenolic ethers (anethole) and monoterpenes. Fennel has an affinity for Liver, Spleen, Stomach and Kidney meridians, and is warming. Can be used for Cold in the Liver and Stomach Channels with symptoms of abdominal pain, constipation, or difficulty with urination or menstruation. It warms the Middle Heater to promote digestion and strengthens the Kidney and Ming Men Fire (willpower).

SPEARMINT *(Mentha spicata)*
Family: Lamiaceae; can increase metabolism, stimulate the gallbladder; has been used for digestive disorders, as well as release of emotional blocks. High in ketones (carvone). Cooling Spearmint has an affinity for the Lung and Liver meridians and promotes Wei qi movement to relieve muscular and digestive spasms, as well as clears Wind Heat.

COLON AND DIGESTION VRT:
Tuning Fork Intervals

Microtone

Om/Pluto — Microtone, highly dissonant, penetrates deep into the body structure to a cellular level, breaks down resistance to change, unconscious and shadow self level. Pluto rules the elimination of toxic wastes from the body, and assists in all bowel disharmonies.

Fifth, 2:3

High Om/High Earth Day — highly energetic, full of movement, intense propelling energy, joyful. Also considered to be an Augmented 4th or Diminished 5th. This interval has also been called Crux Ansata, a transition point where spirit is redeemed from matter. This interval is the most fundamental one to build energy and eliminate fatigue. We use it near the end of the session, when one's energetic stores need to be nourished and consolidated.

HEART AND CIRCULATION
Vibrational Raindrop Technique
QUICK REFERENCE RAINDROP OUTLINE

Forks:		Essential Oils	
Low Om	High Om	Valor®	Clove
Om x 2	**High Uranus**	Oregano	Aroma Life®
Sun	**High Sun**	Thyme	Cypress
Zodiac Platonic Earth	**Angelic Sun**	Goldenrod	Nutmeg
Venus		White Angelica	

1. **Facilitator: Apply White Angelica to self on shoulders, back of neck, thymus.**
   Apply Om Unison to self at CV-4 (Origin Pass) for grounding.

2. **HAVE CLIENT LIE FACE UP. ESTABLISH ENERGY BALANCE:**
   Listen to Om Unison (2 Om forks) (hold tuning forks at least 6" from client's ears).
   VALOR®: Rub on Shoulders (1-2 drops/shoulder) and Feet (1-2 drops/foot),
   R hand/R foot, L hand/L foot; R hand/R shoulder, L hand/L shoulder.
   Hold until you feel the energy balance left and right.
   Apply Om Unison (1 Om fork to the sole of each foot) at KI-1 (Gushing Spring).

3. **VIBRATIONAL VITA FLEX on Spinal Reflex Area of Feet** (1-3 drops each oil to each foot)

VALOR®	**OREGANO**	**THYME**
GOLDENROD	**CLOVE**	**AROMA LIFE®**
CYPRESS	**NUTMEG**	

   Apply the Om Octave (Om and Low Om forks) with Low Om at CV-4 (Origin Pass) on the abdomen four finger-widths below the umbilicus, and Om at CV-17 (Chest Center) in the center of the chest level with the 4th rib. Then apply the Om Octave (Om and Low Om forks) with Low Om at CV-17 (Chest Center) and Om at GV-24.5 (Yin Tang) between the eyebrows.
   • HAVE CLIENT ROLL OVER TO A FACE DOWN POSITION

4. **OREGANO:** Raindrop V-6 (6" above) 4-6 drops from sacrum to atlas.
   Raindrop (6" above) 1-2 drops Oregano from sacrum to atlas.
   Feather stroke 3" straight up spine. Repeat with 6" then 12" strokes.
   THYME: Raindrop (6" above) 1-2 drops Thyme from sacrum to atlas.
   Feather stroke 3" straight up spine. Repeat with 6" then 12" strokes.
   Feather straight to sides in each position.
   Feather with full length strokes up and out, off the shoulders.
   Apply the Solar 7th (Low Om and Sun forks) with the Low Om on GV-2 (Low Back Shu) at base of sacrum and Sun fork on GV-11 (Spirit Path) below T-5. Then apply Low Om on GV-11 and Sun on GV-20 on the crown of the head.

5. GOLDENROD, CLOVE, and AROMA LIFE®

> Raindrop and feather each oil on spine, as in Step 4 (Oregano).
> Finger circles (after all three oils are applied).

Apply Zodiac Platonic 3rd (Om and Zodiac Platonic Earth forks) wherever muscle knots are found. Apply the Zodiac Platonic 3rd to the bank of muscles next to the spine, one side at a time. Walk up this band with the forks, moving about 2-3" each time, with Om closer to the feet and Zodiac Platonic Earth closer to the head. When completed, apply Om at the bottom of the band and Zodiac Platonic Earth at the top of the band.

6. CYPRESS

> Sprinkle (6" above) from sacrum to atlas.
> Feather stroke 3" straight up spine. Repeat with 6" then 12" strokes.
> Thumb Vitaflex up spine.
> Saw Maneuver up spine.
> Stretch and Quiver up spine.

Apply the Venus Minor 6th (Om and Venus forks) on the Huato Jiaji points up the spine from sacrum to base of skull, alternating the Venus and Om forks on either side of the spine up to the atlas, then hold both forks at the crown of the head, GV-20.

7. ORTHO EASE®

> Apply to entire back, followed by large circles with palms.
> Palm Slide up & down the back. Apply more Ortho Ease® if needed.

Sound the High Solar 7th (High Om and Angelic Sun forks) and move in a DN-8 figure over the client, from feet to crown, then back down off the feet.

8. VALOR®

> Sprinkle (6" above) from sacrum to atlas.
> Feather stroke 3" straight up spine. Repeat with 6" then 12" strokes.
> Arched feather stroke 3" straight up spine. Repeat with 6" then 12" strokes.
> Feather with full length strokes up and out, off the shoulders.

Sound the High Sun Octave (High Sun and Angelic Sun forks) and move in a DN-8 figure over the client, from feet to crown, then down off the feet.

9. NUTMEG (Use sparingly: 1-2 drops)

> Raindrop (6" above) 1-2 drops from sacrum to atlas. Feather as with Valor.

10. WARM COMPRESS

Apply hot compress; cool compress for MS clients.

Sound the High Uranus 5th (High Om and High Uranus forks), move in a DN-8 figure over the client from feet to crown, then down off the feet.

Apply the Om Octave (Om and Low Om forks) to the sole of each foot at KI-1 (Gushing Spring).

11 & 12   EVALUATE AND GIVE WATER

HEART AND CIRCULATION VRT:
Essential Oils

All of the Systems-specific Vibrational Raindrop Technique protocol use Valor, oregano and thyme as the core three oils to open and close Vibrational Raindrop Technique (EDOR, 4th Ed, page 299). Basil, marjoram, wintergreen, cypress and peppermint are replaced with oils more specific to the body system being treated. Details on specific oils used to focus on the Heart/Circulation system are included below.

GOLDENROD *(Solidago canadensis)*

Family: Asteraceae (aster-daisy family), is a diuretic, anti-hypertensive. Contains 30-55% monoterpenes, 24-35% sesquiterpenes which may assist in restoring proper cellular programming to restore health and maintain wellness.

Slightly cooling, Goldenrod has an affinity with the Kidney and Spleen meridians. Its actions are similar to Cypress, in that it astringes fluid discharge that results from leakage of qi, such as urine, sweat, bedwetting, or diarrhea.

NUTMEG *(Myristica fragrans)*

Family: Myristicaceae (myrtle family), has potent anti-inflammatory (ORAC 158,100), and anticoagulant properties. Also used for its adrenal cortex-like activity to help support the adrenal glands for increased energy. Contains 55-80% monoterpenes which may assist in restoring proper cellular programming.

Warming Nutmeg has an affinity to the Liver, Spleen, and Large Intestine meridians.
It is useful for Deficient Spleen symptoms of chronic diarrhea, scant and painful menses, and impotence. It will warm and regulate qi in the Middle Heater to assist with symptoms of nausea and vomiting.

AROMA LIFE®

(Contains helichrysum, ylang ylang, marjoram and cypress); improves cardiovascular, lymphatic and circulatory systems; lowers high blood pressure and reduces stress.

CYPRESS *(Cupressus sempervirens)*

Family: Cupressaceae (cypress family) is antimicrobial. Supportive of the circulatory and lymphatic systems. Stimulates the body's natural white corpuscle production. 76% monoterpenes and 14% sesquiterpenes which may assist in restoring proper cellular programming to restore health and maintain wellness.

Slightly cooling, Cypress has an affinity for Lung, Spleen, and Kidney meridians. It astringes fluid discharge that results from leakage of qi, such as urine, sweat, or diarrhea. Cypress ascends Spleen qi to upbear prolapse, hemorrhoids, and varicose veins. Finally, it is very helpful to clear Lung heat and assists the Kidney to grasp Lung qi in wheezing and bedwetting.

CLOVE *(Syzygium aromaticum)*

Family: Myristicaceae (myrtle family), anti-aging, cardiovascular disease, anticoagulant properties. Contains 70-85% phenols which cleanse cellular receptor sites.

Hot by nature, Clove has an affinity for the Spleen, Stomach and Kidney meridians. It can be used to warm the Kidneys to treat bone, teeth, and impotence; to warm the interior/expel Cold in the Stomach and Spleen, which will assist digestive problems and abdominal pain. Clove also improves thyroid and immune function by strengthening Deficient Spleen and Kidney qi.

HEART AND CIRCULATION VRT:
Tuning Fork Intervals

Fifth, 2:3

High Om/High Uranus – the Electrical Fifth; opens with the electrical charge of transformation, can shatter pre-existing conceptions and embodies the energy of freedom and independence. Mentally transformative, illuminating, inventive and break-through ideas. Uranus governs the electrical activity of the nervous system, and can calm and balance it.

Minor 7th, 5:9

Om/High Sun – harsh but more distant, less emotional than the Minor 2nd (its inversion). Strong, warm energy, this interval is used near the completion of Raindrop to assist in deletion of old, redundant and useless information so changes can occur and a new order can be achieved.

Minor 6th, 5:8

Om/Venus – mellow sense of longing; tonifies, nourishes beauty, harmony and creative passion but has a quality of inconstancy, desire and yearning for completion. This interval is used for assisting with bone density and circulation.

Octave, 1:2

High Sun/Angelic Sun – very warming and energizing Octave, bright sunshine on a cloudy day. This interval is used after the Ortho Ease rub to allow an interval of basking in the fullness of one's highest energy and well-being.

HORMONE BALANCE - FEMALE
Vibrational Raindrop Technique
QUICK REFERENCE RAINDROP OUTLINE

Forks:		Essential Oils	
Low Om	High Om	Valor®	Fleabane
Om x 2	High Jupiter	Oregano	EndoFlex®
Sun	**High Saturn**	Thyme	Clary Sage
Zodiac Platonic Earth	**High Venus**	Dragon Time®	Peppermint
New Synodic Moon		White Angelica	

1. **Facilitator: Apply White Angelica to self on shoulders, back of neck, thymus.**
Apply Om Unison to self at CV-4 (Origin Pass) for grounding.

2. **HAVE CLIENT LIE FACE UP. ESTABLISH ENERGY BALANCE:**
    Listen to Om Unison (2 Om forks) (hold tuning forks at least 6" from client's ears).
    VALOR®: Rub on Shoulders (1-2 drops/shoulder) and Feet (1-2 drops/foot),
    R hand/R foot, L hand/L foot; R hand/R shoulder, L hand/L shoulder.
    Hold until you feel the energy balance left and right.
    Apply Om Unison (1 Om fork to the sole of each foot) at KI-1 (Gushing Spring).

3. **VIBRATIONAL VITA FLEX on Spinal Reflex Area of Feet** (1-3 drops each oil to each foot)
    VALOR®
    OREGANO
    THYME
    DRAGON TIME®
    FLEABANE
    ENDOFLEX®
    CLARY SAGE
    PEPPERMINT
Apply the Om Octave (Om and Low Om forks) with Low Om at CV-4 (Origin Pass) on the abdomen four finger-widths below the umbilicus, and Om at CV-17 (Chest Center) in the center of the chest level with the 4th rib. Then apply the Om Octave (Om and Low Om forks) with Low Om at CV-17 (Chest Center) and Om at GV-24.5 (Yin Tang) between the eyebrows.
    • **HAVE CLIENT ROLL OVER TO A FACE DOWN POSITION**

4. **OREGANO:** Raindrop V-6 (6" above) 4-6 drops from sacrum to atlas.
    Raindrop (6" above) 1-2 drops Oregano from sacrum to atlas.
    Feather stroke 3" straight up spine. Repeat with 6" then 12" strokes.
    THYME: Raindrop (6" above) 1-2 drops Thyme from sacrum to atlas.

Feather stroke 3" straight up spine. Repeat with 6" then 12" strokes.

Feather straight to sides in each position.

Feather with full length strokes up and out, off the shoulders.

Apply the Solar 7th (Low Om and Sun forks) with the Low Om on GV-2 (Low Back Shu) at base of sacrum and Sun fork on GV-11 (Spirit Path) below T-5. Then apply Low Om on GV-11 and Sun on GV-20 on the crown of the head.

5. DRAGON TIME®, FLEABANE, and ENDOFLEX®

Raindrop and feather each oil on spine, as in Step 4 (Oregano).

Finger circles (after all three oils are applied).

Apply Zodiac Platonic 3rd (Om and Zodiac Platonic Earth forks) wherever muscle knots are found. Apply the Zodiac Platonic 3rd to the bank of muscles next to the spine, one side at a time. Walk up this band with the forks, moving about 2-3" each time, with Om closer to the feet and Zodiac Platonic Earth closer to the head. When completed, apply Om at the bottom of the band and Zodiac Platonic Earth at the top of the band.

6. CLARY SAGE

Sprinkle (6" above) from sacrum to atlas.

Feather stroke 3" straight up spine. Repeat with 6" then 12" strokes.

Thumb Vitaflex up spine.

Saw Maneuver up spine.

Stretch and Quiver up spine.

Apply New Synodic Moon 5th (Om and New Synodic Moon forks) on the Huato Jiaji points up the spine from sacrum to base of skull, alternating the New Synodic Moon and Om forks on either side of the spine up to the atlas, then hold both forks at the crown of the head, GV-20.

7. ORTHO EASE®

Apply to entire back, followed by large circles with palms.

Palm Slide up & down the back. Apply more Ortho Ease® if needed.

Sound the High Jupiter 4th (High Om and High Jupiter forks) and move in a DN-8 figure over the client, from feet to crown, then back down off the feet.

8. VALOR®

Sprinkle (6" above) from sacrum to atlas.

Feather stroke 3" straight up spine. Repeat with 6" then 12" strokes.

Arched feather stroke 3" straight up spine. Repeat with 6" then 12" strokes.

Feather with full length strokes up and out, off the shoulders.

Sound the High Saturn minor 2nd (High Om and High Saturn forks) and move in a DN-8 figure over the client, from feet to crown, then down off the feet.

9. PEPPERMINT (Use sparingly: 1-2 drops)
      Raindrop (6" above) 1-2 drops from sacrum to atlas. Feather as with Valor.

10. HOT COMPRESS (For MS clients use a Cold Pack)
      Apply hot compress; cool compress for MS clients.
Sound the High Venus minor 6th (High Om and High Venus forks), move in a DN-8 figure over the client from feet to crown, then down off the feet.

Apply the Om Octave (Om and Low Om forks) to the sole of each foot at KI-1 (Gushing Spring).

11 & 12   EVALUATE AND GIVE WATER

HORMONE BALANCE - FEMALE VRT:
Essential Oils

All of the Systems-specific Vibrational Raindrop Technique protocol use Valor, oregano and thyme as the core three oils to open and close Vibrational Raindrop Technique (EDOR, 4th Ed, page 299). Basil, marjoram, wintergreen, cypress and peppermint are replaced with oils more specific to the body system being treated. Details about the specific oils used to focus on the Hormone Balance – Female system are included below.

DRAGON TIME®
(Contains clary sage, blue yarrow, lavender, jasmine, fennel and marjoram); relieves PMS symptoms as well as cramping, irregular periods and mood swings caused by hormonal imbalance.

FLEABANE *(Conyza canadensis)*
Family: Asteraceae or Compositae (daisy); is hormone-like, antirheumatic, antispasmodic and a cardiovascular dilator. Contains 63-83% monoterpenes. With an affinity for the Kidney, Lung and Spleen meridians, Fleabane is cool in nature. It expels Hot Phlegm and Nourishes Yin, so use it for bronchitis and fevers, as well as a diuretic for edema.

ENDO FLEX®
(Contains spearmint, sage, geranium, myrtle, German Chamomile and nutmeg); amplifies metabolism and vitality, and creates hormonal balance.

CLARY SAGE *(Salvia sclarea)*
Family: Lamiaceae (mint); naturally raises estrogen and progesterone levels, antidiabetic, antifungal, cholesterol-reducing. Very calming and stress-relieving; enhances dreams. Contains 50-78% esters, up to 27% alcohols and up to 14% sesquiterpenes.

Cooling Clary Sage has an affinity for the Liver, Heart and Kidney meridians. It cools Heat in the Blood and Empty Fire with symptoms of night sweats, hot flashes and insomnia. Tonifies Heart Blood and Yin deficiency to resolve anxiety and insomnia.

PEPPERMINT *(Mentha piperita)*
CT menthol – Family: Lamiaceae supports digestive system, respiratory system, and nervous system. Has been used for headaches. Research has shown that inhaling peppermint improves concentration and mental retention. Detoxing to the liver. A synergistic oil that supports and improves the beneficial actions of other oils used in conjunction. High in phenolics, but contains 9% sesquiterpenes.

Peppermint has an affinity for the Lung and Liver meridians with its cooling energy. Clears Wind Heat of headaches, fever, sore throat, and dry cough, as well as regulates Liver qi to promote menstruation, and decongest the Liver/PMS. It also promotes the movement of Wei qi.

HORMONE BALANCE - FEMALE VRT:
Tuning Fork Intervals

Minor Second, 15:16

High Om/High Saturn — semitone and somewhat dissonant, supports the formation of new boundaries and structures. The Minor Second is the most dissonant of the intervals, and Saturn/Om is more dissonant than Mars/Om. They both represent the applications of energy toward the manifestation of material form, in other words creating matter from spirit. Twin pillars of evolution on the material and spiritual planes. We use this interval near the end of the Raindrop session to consolidate the endocrine and hormonal balancing that has begun with Raindrop.

Fifth, 2:3

Om/New Synodic Moon — calming, relaxing, opening. The New Moon 5th is dispersive for emotional issues, while the Earth Day 5th is better suited to gather and strengthen energy. This interval produces openings on the physical, emotional, and spiritual levels.

Minor Sixth, 5:8

High Om/High Venus — mellow sense of longing; tonifies, nourishes beauty, harmony and creative passion but has a quality of inconstancy, desire and yearning for completion. This interval can assist with reproductive problems and menopausal hormonal imbalances. Relax and know that the cleansing and release are perfect as the Venus energy brings the session to fullness.

HORMONE BALANCE - MALE
Vibrational Raindrop Technique

QUICK REFERENCE RAINDROP OUTLINE

Forks:		Essential Oils	
Low Om	High Om	Valor®	Blue Yarrow
Om x 2	High Jupiter	Oregano	Mister®
Sun	High Saturn	Thyme	Myrtle
Zodiac Platonic Earth	High Venus	Lavender	Peppermint
New Synodic Moon		White Angelica	

1. **Facilitator: Apply White Angelica to self on shoulders, back of neck, thymus.**
   Apply Om Unison to self at CV-4 (Origin Pass) for grounding.

2. **HAVE CLIENT LIE FACE UP. ESTABLISH ENERGY BALANCE:**
   Listen to Om Unison (2 Om forks) (hold tuning forks at least 6" from client's ears).
   VALOR®: Rub on Shoulders (1-2 drops/shoulder) and Feet (1-2 drops/foot),
   R hand/R foot, L hand/L foot; R hand/R shoulder, L hand/L shoulder.
   Hold until you feel the energy balance left and right.
   Apply Om Unison (1 Om fork to the sole of each foot) at KI-1 (Gushing Spring).

3. **VIBRATIONAL VITA FLEX on Spinal Reflex Area of Feet** (1-3 drops each oil to each foot)

VALOR®	OREGANO	THYME
LAVENDER	BLUE YARROW	MISTER®
MYRTLE	PEPPERMINT	

   Apply the Om Octave (Om and Low Om forks) with Low Om at CV-4 (Origin Pass) on the abdomen four finger-widths below the umbilicus, and Om at CV-17 (Chest Center) in the center of the chest level with the 4th rib. Then apply the Om Octave (Om and Low Om forks) with Low Om at CV-17 (Chest Center) and Om at GV-24.5 (Yin Tang) between the eyebrows.
   - **HAVE CLIENT ROLL OVER TO A FACE DOWN POSITION**

4. **OREGANO:** Raindrop V-6 (6" above) 4-6 drops from sacrum to atlas.
   Raindrop (6" above) 1-2 drops Oregano from sacrum to atlas.
   Feather stroke 3" straight up spine. Repeat with 6" then 12" strokes.
   THYME: Raindrop (6" above) 1-2 drops Thyme from sacrum to atlas.
   Feather stroke 3" straight up spine. Repeat with 6" then 12" strokes.
   Feather straight to sides in each position.
   Feather with full length strokes up and out, off the shoulders.
   Apply the Solar 7th (Low Om and Sun forks) with the Low Om on GV-2 (Low Back Shu) at base of sacrum and Sun fork on GV-11 (Spirit Path) below T-5. Then apply Low Om on GV-11 and Sun on GV-20 on the crown of the head.

5. LAVENDER, BLUE YARROW, and MISTER®

Raindrop and feather each oil on spine, as in Step 4 (Oregano).

Finger circles (after all three oils are applied).

Apply Zodiac Platonic 3rd (Om and Zodiac Platonic Earth forks) wherever muscle knots are found. Apply the Zodiac Platonic 3rd to the bank of muscles next to the spine, one side at a time. Walk up this band with the forks, moving about 2-3" each time, with Om closer to the feet and Zodiac Platonic Earth closer to the head. When completed, apply Om at the bottom of the band and Zodiac Platonic Earth at the top of the band.

6. MYRTLE

Sprinkle (6" above) from sacrum to atlas.

Feather stroke 3" straight up spine. Repeat with 6" then 12" strokes.

Thumb Vitaflex up spine.

Saw Maneuver up spine.

Stretch and Quiver up spine.

Apply New Synodic Moon 5th (Om and New Synodic Moon forks) on the Huato Jiaji points up the spine from sacrum to base of skull, alternating the New Synodic Moon and Om forks on either side of the spine up to the atlas, then hold both forks at the crown of the head, GV-20.

7. ORTHO EASE®

Apply to entire back, followed by large circles with palms.

Palm Slide up & down the back. Apply more Ortho Ease® if needed.

Sound the High Jupiter 4th (High Om and High Jupiter forks) and move in a DN-8 figure over the client, from feet to crown, then back down off the feet.

8. VALOR®

Sprinkle (6" above) from sacrum to atlas.

Feather stroke 3" straight up spine. Repeat with 6" then 12" strokes.

Arched feather stroke 3" straight up spine. Repeat with 6" then 12" strokes.

Feather with full length strokes up and out, off the shoulders.

Sound the High Saturn minor 2nd (High Om and High Saturn forks) and move in a DN-8 figure over the client, from feet to crown, then down off the feet.

9. PEPPERMINT (Use sparingly: 1-2 drops)

Raindrop (6" above) 1-2 drops from sacrum to atlas. Feather as with Valor.

10. HOT COMPRESS (For MS clients use a Cold Pack)

Apply hot compress; cool compress for MS clients.

Sound the High Venus minor 6th (High Om and High Venus forks), move in a DN-8 figure over the client from feet to crown, then down off the fe.

Apply the Om Octave (Om and Low Om forks) to the sole of each foot at KI-1 (Gushing Spring) x 3.

11 & 12   EVALUATE AND GIVE WATER

HORMONE BALANCE - MALE VRT:
Essential Oils

All of the Systems-specific Vibrational Raindrop Technique protocol use Valor, oregano and thyme as the core three oils to open and close Vibrational Raindrop Technique (EDOR, 4th Ed, page 299). Basil, marjoram, wintergreen, cypress and peppermint are replaced with oils more specific to the body system being treated. Details about the specific oils used to focus on the Hormone Balance – Male system are included below.

LAVENDER *(Lavandula angustifolia)*
Family: Lamiacea (mint); relaxant, combats excess sebum on skin, calming both physically and emotionally. Contains 30-58% alcohols, 26-52% esters.

Cooling Lavender has an affinity for the Lung, Liver, and Pericardium meridians. Use it for Liver Qi Stagnation to promote the smooth flow of Liver qi and resolve headaches, muscle spasms and tightness. Also indicated to Calm the Shen and resolves symptoms of irritability, restlessness and high blood pressure (Liver and Heart Fire).

BLUE YARROW *(Achillea millefolium)*
Family: Asteraceae or Compositae (daisy); considered sacred by the Chinese who recognize the harmony of the Yin and Yang energies within it; where heaven meets earth.

Yarrow is cold in nature with an affinity for the Lung, Liver, and Spleen channels. It is useful for Liver Qi Stagnation symptoms of muscle spasm, wind-bi (radiating pain), indecisiveness and itching skin. It will also release the Exterior by promoting diaphoresis and expelling Phlegm.

MISTER®
(Contains blue yarrow, sage, myrtle fennel, lavender and peppermint); helps to decongest the prostate and promote greater male hormonal balance.

MYRTLE *(Myrtus communis)*
Family: Myrtaceae (myrtle); normalizes hormonal imbalances, thyroid problems, prostate problems, and muscle spasms. Contains 31- 48% oxides, 30-45% monoterpenes.

Dry and cool, Myrtle clears Lung Heat and astringes leakage of qi and Blood such as sweating, bleeding, diarrhea, and hemorrhoids. It is calming as a nervine.

PEPPERMINT *(Mentha piperita)*

CT menthol – Family: Lamiaceae (mint) supports digestive system, respiratory system, and nervous system. Has been used for headaches. Research has shown that inhaling peppermint improves concentration and mental retention. Detoxing to the liver. A synergistic oil that supports and improves the beneficial actions of other oils used in conjunction. High in phenolics, but contains 9% sesquiterpenes.

Peppermint has an affinity for the Lung and Liver meridians with its cooling energy. Clears Wind Heat of headaches, fever, sore throat, and dry cough. Peppermint also regulates Liver qi which, in women, promotes menstruation, and decongest the Liver/PMS. It also promotes the movement of Wei qi.

HORMONE BALANCE - MALE VRT:
Tuning Fork Intervals

Minor Second, 15:16

High Om/High Saturn – semitone and somewhat dissonant, supports the formation of new boundaries and structures. The Minor Second is the most dissonant of the intervals, and Saturn/Om is more dissonant than Mars/Om. They both represent the applications of energy toward the manifestation of material form, in other words creating matter from spirit. Twin pillars of evolution on the material and spiritual planes. We use this interval near the end of the Raindrop session to consolidate the endocrine and hormonal balancing that has begun with Raindrop.

Fifth, 2:3

Om/New Synodic Moon – calming, relaxing, opening. The New Moon 5th is dispersive for emotional issues, while the Earth Day 5th is better suited to gather and strengthen energy. This interval produces openings on the physical, emotional, and spiritual levels.

Minor Sixth, 5:8

High Om/High Venus – mellow sense of longing; tonifies, nourishes beauty, harmony and creative passion but has a quality of inconstancy, desire and yearning for completion. This interval can assist with reproductive problems and menopausal hormonal imbalances. Relax and know that the cleansing and.release are perfect as the Venus energy brings the session to fullness.

JOINTS AND BONES
Vibrational Raindrop Technique
QUICK REFERENCE RAINDROP OUTLINE

Forks:		Essential Oils	
Low Om	High Om	Valor®	Wintergreen
Om x 2	High Full Sidereal Moon	Oregano	Panaway®
Sun	High Jupiter	Thyme	Spruce
Zodiac Platonic Earth	High Mars	Helichrysum	Peppermint
Mars	**Mercury**	White Angelica	
Saturn			

1. **Facilitator: Apply White Angelica to self on shoulders, back of neck, thymus.**
   Apply Om Unison to self at CV-4 (Origin Pass) for grounding.

2. **HAVE CLIENT LIE FACE UP. ESTABLISH ENERGY BALANCE:**
   Listen to Om Unison (2 Om forks) (hold tuning forks at least 6" from client's ears).
   VALOR®: Rub on Shoulders (1-2 drops/shoulder) and Feet (1-2 drops/foot),
   R hand/R foot, L hand/L foot; R hand/R shoulder, L hand/L shoulder.
   Hold until you feel the energy balance left and right.
   Apply Om Unison (1 Om fork to the sole of each foot) at KI-1 (Gushing Spring).

3. **VIBRATIONAL VITA FLEX on Spinal Reflex Area of Feet** (1-3 drops each oil to each foot)

VALOR®	**OREGANO**	**THYME**
HELICHRYSUM	**WINTERGREEN**	**PANAWAY®**
SPRUCE	**PEPPERMINT**	

   Apply the Om Octave (Om and Low Om forks) with Low Om at CV-4 (Origin Pass) on the abdomen four finger-widths below the umbilicus, and Om at CV-17 (Chest Center) in the center of the chest level with the 4th rib. Then apply the Om Octave (Om and Low Om forks) with Low Om at CV-17 (Chest Center) and Om at GV-24.5 (Yin Tang) between the eyebrows.
   - **HAVE CLIENT ROLL OVER TO A FACE DOWN POSITION**

4. **OREGANO:** Raindrop V-6 (6" above) 4-6 drops from sacrum to atlas.
   Raindrop (6" above) 1-2 drops Oregano from sacrum to atlas.
   Feather stroke 3" straight up spine. Repeat with 6" then 12" strokes.
   THYME: Raindrop (6" above) 1-2 drops Thyme from sacrum to atlas.
   Feather stroke 3" straight up spine. Repeat with 6" then 12" strokes.
   Feather straight to sides in each position.
   Feather with full length strokes up and out, off the shoulders.
   Apply the Solar 7th (Low Om and Sun forks) with the Low Om on GV-2 (Low Back Shu) at base of sacrum and Sun fork on GV-11 (Spirit Path) below T-5. Then apply Low Om on GV-11 and Sun on GV-20 on the crown of the head.

5. HELICHRYSUM, WINTERGREEN, and PANAWAY®

Raindrop and feather each oil on spine, as in Step 4 (Oregano).

Finger circles (after all three oils are applied).

Apply Zodiac Platonic 3rd (Om and Zodiac Platonic Earth forks) wherever muscle knots are found. Apply the Zodiac Platonic 3rd to the bank of muscles next to the spine, one side at a time. Walk up this band with the forks, moving about 2-3" each time, with Om closer to the feet and Zodiac Platonic Earth closer to the head. When completed, apply Om at the bottom of the band and Zodiac Platonic Earth at the top of the band.

6. SPRUCE

Sprinkle (6" above) from sacrum to atlas.

Feather stroke 3" straight up spine. Repeat with 6" then 12" strokes.

Thumb Vitaflex up spine.

Saw Maneuver up spine.

Stretch and Quiver up spine.

Apply the Om Unison (two Om forks) on the Huato Jiaji points up the spine from sacrum to base of skull, then hold both forks at the crown of the head, GV-20.

Apply the appropriate interval around the joint/area in question: For example, use the Mercury Microtone (Om and Mercury forks) for the shoulders, the Saturn minor 2nd (Om and Saturn forks) for the knees, and the Mars minor 2nd (Om and Mars forks) for general muscle tension.

7. ORTHO EASE®

Apply to entire back, followed by large circles with palms.

Palm Slide up & down the back. Apply more Ortho Ease® if needed.

Sound the High Jupiter 4th (High Om and High Jupiter forks) and move in a DN-8 figure over the client, from feet to crown, then back down off the feet.

8. VALOR®

Sprinkle (6" above) from sacrum to atlas.

Feather stroke 3" straight up spine. Repeat with 6" then 12" strokes.

Arched feather stroke 3" straight up spine. Repeat with 6" then 12" strokes.

Feather with full length strokes up and out, off the shoulders.

Sound the High Mars minor 2nd (High Om and High Mars forks) and move in a DN-8 figure over the client, from feet to crown, then down off the feet.

9. PEPPERMINT (Use sparingly: 1-2 drops)

Raindrop (6" above) 1-2 drops from sacrum to atlas. Feather as with Valor.

10. WARM COMPRESS

Apply hot compress; cool compress for MS clients.

Sound the High Full Sidereal Moon Major 6th (High Om and High Full Sidereal Moon forks), move in a DN-8 figure over the client from feet to crown, then down off the feet.

Apply the Om Octave (Om and Low Om forks) to the sole of each foot at KI-1 (Gushing Spring).

11 & 12   EVALUATE AND GIVE WATER

JOINTS AND BONES VRT:
Essential Oils

All of the Systems-specific Vibrational Raindrop Technique protocol use Valor, oregano and thyme as the core three oils to open and close Vibrational Raindrop Technique (EDOR, 4th Ed, page 299). Basil, marjoram, wintergreen, cypress and peppermint are replaced with oils more specific to the body system being treated. Details about the specific oils used to focus on the Joints/Bones system are included below.

HELICHRYSUM *(Helichrysum italicum)*

Family: Asteraceae (daisy); antispasmodic, detoxifier, regenerates nerves. Contains 28-60% esters, 16 22% ketones and 10-20% sesquiterpenes.

Cooling Helichrysum has an affinity for Lung and Liver meridians. It Clears Damp Heat Bi Obstruction and is excellent for breaking up fibrotic tissue. Can be very useful during a drug or chemical detox since it addresses Liver Fire leading to Liver Blood Stasis.

WINTERGREEN *(Gaultheria procumbens)*

Family: Ericaceae (heather) supports joints and skeletal structure. Composition of both of this oil is more than 80% methyl salicylate (a phenolic ester) which has a cortisone-like effect in that it may stimulate the body's own production of natural cortisone which has none of the untoward side-effects of synthetic cortisone. Also has analgesic properties inasmuch as its chemical structure is similar to that of aspirin.

Warming by nature and with an affinity for Bladder and Kidney meridians, Wintergreen expels Wind Damp Cold Bi Obstruction, so finds excellent application along the spine for chronic back problems.

SPRUCE *(Picea mariana)*

Family Pinaceae (pine); used for arthritis, rheumatism, sciatica, and lumbago. Used by the Lakota to strengthen their ability to communicate with the Great Spirit. Traditionally believed to possess the frequency of prosperity. Contains 45-55% monoterpenes, 30-37% esters.

Spruce has an affinity for the Lung and Kidney meridians, and is warming. It is indicated for Deficient Kidney Yang and will expel wind Cold Bi Obstruction of back pain. Use for coughing and asthma to descend Lung Qi to the Kidneys.

PANAWAY®

(Contains helichrysum, wintergreen, clove, and peppermint); reduces pain and inflammation, increases circulation and accelerates healing. Relieves swelling and pain from arthritis, sprains, muscle spasms and bruises.

PEPPERMINT *(Mentha piperita)*

CT menthol – Family: Lamiaceae, supports digestive system, respiratory system, and nervous system. Has been used for headaches. Research has shown that inhaling peppermint improves concentration and mental retention. Detoxing to the liver. A synergistic oil that supports and improves the beneficial actions of other oils used in conjunction. High in phenolics, but contains 9% sesquiterpenes.

Peppermint has an affinity for the Lung and Liver meridians with its cooling energy. Clears Wind Heat of headaches, fever, sore throat, and dry cough, as well as regulates Liver qi to promote menstruation, and decongest the Liver/PMS. It also promotes the movement of Wei qi.

JOINTS AND BONES VRT:
Tuning Fork Intervals

Microtone

Om/Mercury – creates a great deal of movement and dissonance; volatile, going between the cracks, mental illumination and communication. Mercury has an affinity with the nervous system and communication of all kinds. Use this interval for all problems with the shoulders, arms and hands, especially if the nerves are involved.

Minor Second, 15:16

Om/Mars – harsh; carrier of considerable energetic potential, propels the mind, body and spirit into action with power and initiative to remove obstacles. This interval is used all muscle problems such as atrophy, hypertrophy, spasm, and influences the proper functioning of the muscle system. This interval is also used near the end of the journey, when we need to mobilize our energies and courage to move and release the unnecessary burdens that we carry.

Om/Saturn – semitone and somewhat dissonant, supports the formation of new boundaries and structures. The Minor Second is the most dissonant of the intervals, and Om/Saturn is more dissonant than Om/Mars. They both represent the applications of energy toward the manifestation of material form, in other words creating matter from spirit. Twin pillars of evolution on the material and spiritual planes. Use this interval for all problems with skeleton, arthritis, chronic subluxations, cartilage, ligaments and fascia.

LIVER
Vibrational Raindrop Technique
QUICK REFERENCE RAINDROP OUTLINE

Forks:		Essential Oils	
Low Om	High Om	Valor®	German Chamomile
Om x 2	High Full Sidereal Moon	Oregano	Juvaflex®
Sun	**High Pluto**	Thyme	Ledum
Zodiac Platonic Earth	**High Zodiac Pl Earth**	Carrot Seed	Peppermint
Jupiter		White Angelica	

1. **Facilitator: Apply White Angelica to self on shoulders, back of neck, thymus.**
   Apply Om Unison to self at CV-4 (Origin Pass) for grounding.

2. **HAVE CLIENT LIE FACE UP. ESTABLISH ENERGY BALANCE:**
   Listen to Om Unison (2 Om forks) (hold tuning forks at least 6" from client's ears).
   VALOR®: Rub on Shoulders (1-2 drops/shoulder) and Feet (1-2 drops/foot),
   R hand/R foot, L hand/L foot; R hand/R shoulder, L hand/L shoulder.
   Hold until you feel the energy balance left and right.
   Apply Om Unison (1 Om fork to the sole of each foot) at KI-1 (Gushing Spring).

3. **VIBRATIONAL VITA FLEX on Spinal Reflex Area of Feet** (1-3 drops each oil to each foot)
VALOR®	**OREGANO**	**THYME**
CARROT SEED	**GERMAN CHAMOMILE**	**JUVAFLEX®**
LEDUM	**PEPPERMINT**	

   Apply the Om Octave (Om and Low Om forks) with Low Om at CV-4 (Origin Pass) on the abdomen four finger-widths below the umbilicus, and Om at CV-17 (Chest Center) in the center of the chest level with the 4th rib. Then apply the Om Octave (Om and Low Om forks) with Low Om at CV-17 (Chest Center) and Om at GV-24.5 (Yin Tang) between the eyebrows.
   - **HAVE CLIENT ROLL OVER TO A FACE DOWN POSITION**

4. **OREGANO:** Raindrop V-6 (6" above) 4-6 drops from sacrum to atlas.
   Raindrop (6" above) 1-2 drops Oregano from sacrum to atlas.
   Feather stroke 3" straight up spine. Repeat with 6" then 12" strokes.
   THYME: Raindrop (6" above) 1-2 drops Thyme from sacrum to atlas.
   Feather stroke 3" straight up spine. Repeat with 6" then 12" strokes.
   Feather straight to sides in each position.
   Feather with full length strokes up and out, off the shoulders.
   Apply the Solar 7th (Low Om and Sun forks) with the Low Om on GV-2 (Low Back Shu) at base of sacrum and Sun fork on GV-11 (Spirit Path) below T-5. Then apply Low Om on GV-11 and Sun on GV-20 on the crown of the head.

5. **CARROT SEED, GERMAN CHAMOMILE, and JUVAFLEX®**

   Raindrop and feather each oil on spine, as in Step 4 (Oregano).

   Finger circles (after all three oils are applied).

   Apply Zodiac Platonic 3rd (Om and Zodiac Platonic Earth forks) wherever muscle knots are found. Apply the Zodiac Platonic 3rd to the bank of muscles next to the spine, one side at a time. Walk up this band with the forks, moving about 2-3" each time, with Om closer to the feet and Zodiac Platonic Earth closer to the head. When completed, apply Om at the bottom of the band and Zodiac Platonic Earth at the top of the band.

6. **LEDUM**

   Sprinkle (6" above) from sacrum to atlas.

   Feather stroke 3" straight up spine. Repeat with 6" then 12" strokes.

   Thumb Vitaflex up spine.

   Saw Maneuver up spine.

   Stretch and Quiver up spine.

   Apply the Jupiter 4th (Om and Jupiter forks) on the Huato Jiaji points up the spine from sacrum to base of skull, alternating Jupiter and Om forks on either side of the spine up to the atlas, then hold both forks at the crown of the head, GV-20.

7. **ORTHO EASE®**

   Apply to entire back, followed by large circles with palms.

   Palm Slide up & down the back. Apply more Ortho Ease® if needed.

   Sound the High Zodiac Platonic Earth 3rd (High Om and High Zodiac Platonic Earth forks) and move in a DN-8 figure over the client, from feet to crown, then back down off the feet.

8. **VALOR®**

   Sprinkle (6" above) from sacrum to atlas.

   Feather stroke 3" straight up spine. Repeat with 6" then 12" strokes.

   Arched feather stroke 3" straight up spine. Repeat with 6" then 12" strokes.

   Feather with full length strokes up and out, off the shoulders.

   Sound the High Pluto microtone (High Om and High Pluto forks) and move in a DN-8 figure over the client, from feet to crown, then down off the feet.

9. **PEPPERMINT** (Use sparingly: 1-2 drops)

   Raindrop (6" above) 1-2 drops from sacrum to atlas . Feather as with Valor.

10. WARM COMPRESS

Apply hot compress; cool compress for MS clients.

Sound the High Full Sidereal Moon Major 6th (High Om and High Full Sidereal Moon forks), move in a DN-8 figure over the client from feet to crown, then down off the feet.

Apply the Om Octave (Om and Low Om forks) to the sole of each foot at KI-1 (Gushing Spring).

11 & 12   EVALUATE AND GIVE WATER

LIVER VRT:
Essential Oils

All of the Systems-specific Vibrational Raindrop Technique protocol use Valor, oregano and thyme as the core three oils to open and close Vibrational Raindrop Technique (EDOR, 4th Ed, page 299). Basil, marjoram, wintergreen, cypress and peppermint are replaced with oils more specific to the body system being treated. Details about the specific oils used to focus on the Liver system are included below.

JUVAFLEX®
Contains geranium, rosemary, Roman Chamomile, fennel, helichrysum and blue tansy); supports liver and lymphatic detoxification, helps break addictions to coffee, drugs, alcohol, tobacco and anger.

GERMAN CHAMOMILE *(Matricaria recutita)*
Family: Asteraceae (daisy); powerful antioxidant (inhibits lipid perosidation), anti-inflammatory, promotes digestion, liver and gallbladder health. Dispels anger, helps release emotions linked to the past. Soothes and clears the mind. Contains 33-57% oxides, 34-60% sesquiterpenes.

Cooling and with an affinity for the Liver and Heart meridians, German Chamomile clears Liver Fire and subdues Liver Wind to assist with headaches, anger outbursts, diaphragmatic construction and muscle cramps. It calms the Shen to reduce anxiety. German Chamomile also harmonizes Liver and its effect on the Stomach with symptoms of IBS, candida, and ulcers.

CARROT SEED *(Daucus carota)*
Family Apiacea (parsley family); traditionally used for kidney and digestive disorders and to relieve liver congestion, and water retention. Contains 29-47% alcohols, 20-24% monoterpenes, 14-18% sesquiterpenes.

Cooling Carrot Seed nourishes Liver Blood and has an affinity for the Liver and Kidney meridians. It is indicated for Deficient Liver Blood symptoms of dry eyes, poor vision, dizziness, and brittle nails. Carrot Seed oil can also regulate the production of thyroxine.

LEDUM *(Ledum groenlandicum)*
Family: Ericaceae (heather family); diuretic, liver-protectant, used for liver problems, hepatitis, fatty liver, obesity and water retention. Contains 30-50% monoterpenes, 13-20% sesquiterpenes.

Cooling in nature, Ledum has an affinity for the Liver and Spleen meridians. Use it for Liver Qi Stagnation to promote the smooth flow of Liver qi and resolve headaches, abdominal pain, and muscle spasms. Also indicated to Calm the Shen and resolves symptoms of irritability, restlessness and high blood pressure (Liver Fire).

PEPPERMINT *(Mentha piperita)*

CT menthol – Family: Lamiaceae supports digestive system, respiratory system, and nervous system. Has been used for headaches. Research has shown that inhaling peppermint improves concentration and mental retention. Detoxing to the liver. A synergistic oil that supports and improves the beneficial actions of other oils used in conjunction. High in phenolics, but contains 9% sesquiterpenes.

Peppermint has an affinity for the Lung and Liver meridians with its cooling energy. Clears Wind Heat of headaches, fever, sore throat, and dry cough, as well as regulates Liver qi to promote menstruation, and decongest the Liver/PMS. It also promotes the movement of Wei qi.

LIVER VRT:
Tuning Fork Intervals

Microtone

High Om/High Pluto – highly dissonant, penetrates deep into the body structure to a cellular level, breaks down resistance to change, unconscious and shadow self level. Disharmony between notes creates desire for resolution. As the Liver is cleansed, toxins can manifest on the skin; this interval helps to bring the toxins to the surface and clear them.

Major Third, 4:5

High Om/High Zodiac Platonic Earth – optimistic, happy; meditative, dispersive or dispelling effect, relieves mental stress, but is especially useful to relieve physical stress. We use this interval to release stagnant Liver energy, which can be seen in problems such as hot flashes, PMS symptoms, headaches, and anger/ frustration issues.

Fourth, 3:4

Om/Jupiter – Perfect Fourth; pure, like church bells; stimulates growth, abundance and expansion. The Fourth is the geometric mean of an Octave. Jupiter has a natural affinity for the Liver which allows it to influence the production of bile, cholesterol, and glycogen production. Jupiter is also associated with the sciatic nerve, the hips and thighs.

LONGEVITY
Vibrational Raindrop Technique
QUICK REFERENCE RAINDROP OUTLINE

Forks:		Essential Oils	
Low Om	High Om	Valor®	Clove
Om x 2	High Full Sidereal Moon	Oregano	Longevity®
Sun	High Jupiter	Thyme	Frankincense
Zodiac Platonic Earth	**High Neptune**	Orange	Peppermint
Earth Day		White Angelica	

1. **Facilitator: Apply White Angelica to self on shoulders, back of neck, thymus.**
   Apply Om Unison to self at CV-4 (Origin Pass) for grounding.

2. **HAVE CLIENT LIE FACE UP. ESTABLISH ENERGY BALANCE:**
   Listen to Om Unison (2 Om forks) (hold tuning forks at least 6" from client's ears).
   VALOR®: Rub on Shoulders (1-2 drops/shoulder) and Feet (1-2 drops/foot),
   R hand/R foot, L hand/L foot; R hand/R shoulder, L hand/L shoulder.
   Hold until you feel the energy balance left and right.
   Apply Om Unison (1 Om fork to the sole of each foot) at KI-1 (Gushing Spring).

3. **VIBRATIONAL VITA FLEX on Spinal Reflex Area of Feet** (1-3 drops each oil to each foot)
VALOR®	OREGANO	THYME
ORANGE	CLOVE	LONGEVITY®
FRANKINCENSE	PEPPERMINT	

   Apply the Om Octave (Om and Low Om forks) with Low Om at CV-4 (Origin Pass) on the abdomen four finger-widths below the umbilicus, and Om at CV-17 (Chest Center) in the center of the chest level with the 4th rib. Then apply the Om Octave (Om and Low Om forks) with Low Om at CV-17 (Chest Center) and Om at GV-24.5 (Yin Tang) between the eyebrows.
   - **HAVE CLIENT ROLL OVER TO A FACE DOWN POSITION**

4. **OREGANO:** Raindrop V-6 (6" above) 4-6 drops from sacrum to atlas.
   Raindrop (6" above) 1-2 drops Oregano from sacrum to atlas.
   Feather stroke 3" straight up spine. Repeat with 6" then 12" strokes.
   THYME: Raindrop (6" above) 1-2 drops Thyme from sacrum to atlas.
   Feather stroke 3" straight up spine. Repeat with 6" then 12" strokes.
   Feather straight to sides in each position.
   Feather with full length strokes up and out, off the shoulders.
   Apply the Solar 7th (Low Om and Sun forks) with the Low Om on GV-2 (Low Back Shu) at base of sacrum and Sun fork on GV-11 (Spirit Path) below T-5. Then apply Low Om on GV-11 and Sun on GV-20 on the crown of the head.

5. ORANGE, CLOVE, and LONGEVITY®

Raindrop and feather each oil on spine, as in Step 4 (Oregano).

Finger circles (after all three oils are applied).

Apply Zodiac Platonic 3rd (Om and Zodiac Platonic Earth forks) wherever muscle knots are found. Apply the Zodiac Platonic 3rd to the bank of muscles next to the spine, one side at a time. Walk up this band with the forks, moving about 2-3" each time, with Om closer to the feet and Zodiac Platonic Earth closer to the head. When completed, apply Om at the bottom of the band and Zodiac Platonic Earth at the top of the band.

6. FRANKINCENSE

Sprinkle (6" above) from sacrum to atlas.

Feather stroke 3" straight up spine. Repeat with 6" then 12" strokes.

Thumb Vitaflex up spine.

Saw Maneuver up spine.

Stretch and Quiver up spine.

Apply the Earth Day Augmented 4th (Om and Earth Day forks) on the Huato Jiaji points up the spine from sacrum to base of skull, alternating the Earth Day and Om forks on either side of the spine up to the atlas, then hold both forks at the crown of the head, GV-20.

7. ORTHO EASE®

Apply to entire back, followed by large circles with palms.

Palm Slide up & down the back. Apply more Ortho Ease® if needed.

Sound the High Jupiter 4th (High Om and High Jupiter forks) and move in a DN-8 figure over the client, from feet to crown, then back down off the feet.

8. VALOR®

Sprinkle (6" above) from sacrum to atlas.

Feather stroke 3" straight up spine. Repeat with 6" then 12" strokes.

Arched feather stroke 3" straight up spine. Repeat with 6" then 12" strokes.

Feather with full length strokes up and out, off the shoulders.

Sound the High Neptune 5th (High Om and High Neptune forks) and move in a DN-8 figure over the client, from feet to crown, then down off the feet.

9. PEPPERMINT (Use sparingly: 1-2 drops)

Raindrop (6" above) 1-2 drops from sacrum to atlas. Feather as with Valor.

10. WARM COMPRESS

Apply hot compress; cool compress for MS clients.

Sound the High Full Sidereal Moon Major 6th (High Om and High Full Sidereal Moon forks), move in a DN-8 *figure over the client from feet to crown, then down off the feet.*

Apply the Om Octave (Om and Low Om forks) to the sole of each foot at KI-1 (Gushing Spring).

11 & 12   EVALUATE AND GIVE WATER

LONGEVITY VRT:
Essential Oils

All of the Systems-specific Vibrational Raindrop Technique protocols use Valor, oregano, and thyme as the core three oils to open and close Vibrational Raindrop Technique (EDOR, 4th Ed, page 299). Basil, marjoram, wintergreen, cypress and peppermint are replaced with oils more specific to the body system being treated. Details about the specific oils used to focus on the Longevity system are included below.

ORANGE *(Citrus sinensis)*

Family: Rutaceae (citrus); boosts immunity, used for arteriosclerosis, hypertension, cancer and fluid retention. Contains over 90% limonene, which has been studied for its ability to combat tumor growth in over 50 clinical studies.

Orange is cooling with an affinity for Lung, Heart, and Stomach meridians. Use it to Release Wind Heat with fever, chills, and cough; Clear Heart Fire with palpitations, hypertension and insomnia; and to Descend Stomach qi to promote peristalsis and clear symptoms of Stomach Fire (indigestion, nausea, IBS).

CLOVE *(Syzygium aromaticum)*

Family: Myrtaceae (myrtle); anti-aging, cardiovascular disease, anticoagulant properties. Contains 70¬85% phenols which cleanse cellular receptor sites. Clove has the highest known antioxidant power as measured by ORAC (Oxygen Radical Absorbent Capacity), a test developed by USDA researchers at Tufts University. Hot by nature, Clove has an affinity for the Spleen, Stomach, and Kidney meridians. It can be used to warm the Kidneys to treat bone, teeth, and impotence; warm the interior to expel Cold in the Stomach and Spleen to treat digestive problems and abdominal pain. Clove also improves thyroid and immune function by strengthening Deficient Spleen and Kidney qi.

LONGEVITY®

(Contains clove, thyme, orange, and frankincense); has the highest antioxidant and DNA-protecting essential oils, promotes longevity and prevents premature aging. Thyme has been shown to dramatically boost glutathione levels in the heart, liver, and brain. The oxidation of fats in the body is directly linked to accelerated aging, and thyme prevents peroxidation of fats found in many vital organs.

FRANKINCENSE *(Boswellia carteri)*

Family: Burseraceae (frankincense); antitumoral, immunostimulant, antidepressant; increases spiritual awareness, promotes meditation, improves attitude. Contains 64-90% monoterpenes, 5-10% sesquiterpenes, which stimulate the limbic system of the brain (the center of memory and emotions), and the hypothalamus, pineal, and pituitary glands.

Slightly cooling and drying, Frankincense has an affinity for the Lung, Heart and Kidney meridians. Use it for Lung Heat with Chest Qi Stasis symptoms of agitation, anxiety and irritability. Clears heat in the Lungs with coughing or wheezing, Stomach with ulcers, and Kidneys with cystitis. It can also reduce swelling and treat non-healing wounds, ulcers, and scars.

PEPPERMINT *(Mentha piperita)*

CT menthol – Family: Lamiaceae; supports digestive system, respiratory system, and nervous system. Has been used for headaches. Research has shown that inhaling peppermint improves concentration and mental retention. Detoxifying to the liver. A synergistic oil that supports and improves the beneficial actions of other oils used in conjunction. High in phenolics, but contains 9% sesquiterpenes.

Peppermint has an affinity for the Lung and Liver meridians with its cooling energy. Clears Wind Heat of headaches, fever, sore throat, and dry cough, as well as regulates Liver qi to promote menstruation, and decongest the Liver/PMS. It also promotes the movement of Wei qi.

LONGEVITY VRT:
Tuning Fork Intervals

Fifth, 2:3

Om/Earth Day – highly energetic, full of movement, intense propelling energy, joyful. Also considered to be an Augmented 4th or Diminished 5th. This interval has also been called Crux Ansata, a transition point where spirit is redeemed from matter. This interval is the most fundamental for building energy and eliminating fatigue. If there is a particular Neuro-Endocrine Center (chakra) that is weak, sound the forks extra times at that level of the spine.

High Om/High Neptune – a near Perfect Fifth, aptly called the Ecstatic Fifth, opens and moves the visionary from transpersonal to transcendental, fulfills the yearning for connection with the Infinite. Because of Neptune's association with the spinal canal and spinal cord, we bring the Raindrop session nearly to completion with this interval in sweeping motions the length of the spine and to the feet.

LUNG
Vibrational Raindrop Technique
QUICK REFERENCE RAINDROP OUTLINE

Forks:		Essential Oils	
Low Om	High Om	Valor®	Melrose®
Om x 2	High Full Sidereal Moon	Oregano	Raven®
Sun	High Jupiter	Thyme	Myrtle
Zodiac Platonic Earth	**High New Synodic Moon**	Eucalyptus Radiata	Ravensara
Full Sidereal Moon		White Angelica	

1. **Facilitator: Apply White Angelica to self on shoulders, back of neck, thymus.**
   Apply Om Unison to self at CV-4 (Origin Pass) for grounding.

2. **HAVE CLIENT LIE FACE UP. ESTABLISH ENERGY BALANCE:**
   Listen to Om Unison (2 Om forks) (hold tuning forks at least 6" from client's ears).
   VALOR®: Rub on Shoulders (1-2 drops/shoulder) and Feet (1-2 drops/foot),
   R hand/R foot, L hand/L foot; R hand/R shoulder, L hand/L shoulder.
   Hold until you feel the energy balance left and right.
   Apply Om Unison (1 Om fork to the sole of each foot) at KI-1 (Gushing Spring).

3. **VIBRATIONAL VITA FLEX on Spinal Reflex Area of Feet** (1-3 drops each oil to each foot)

VALOR®	OREGANO	THYME
EUCALYPTUS RADIATA	MELROSE®	RAVEN®
MYRTLE	RAVENSARA	

   Apply the Om Octave (Om and Low Om forks) with Low Om at CV-4 (Origin Pass) on the abdomen four finger-widths below the umbilicus, and Om at CV-17 (Chest Center) in the center of the chest level with the 4th rib. Then apply the Om Octave (Om and Low Om forks) with Low Om at CV-17 (Chest Center) and Om at GV-24.5 (Yin Tang) between the eyebrows.
   - **HAVE CLIENT ROLL OVER TO A FACE DOWN POSITION**

4. **OREGANO:** Raindrop V-6 (6" above) 4-6 drops from sacrum to atlas.
   Raindrop (6" above) 1-2 drops Oregano from sacrum to atlas.
   Feather stroke 3" straight up spine. Repeat with 6" then 12" strokes.
   THYME: Raindrop (6" above) 1-2 drops Thyme from sacrum to atlas.
   Feather stroke 3" straight up spine. Repeat with 6" then 12" strokes.
   Feather straight to sides in each position.
   Feather with full length strokes up and out, off the shoulders.
   Apply the Solar 7th (Low Om and Sun forks) with the Low Om on GV-2 (Low Back Shu) at base of sacrum and Sun fork on GV-11 (Spirit Path) below T-5. Then apply Low Om on GV-11 and Sun on GV-20 on the crown of the head.

5. EUCALYPTUS RADIATA, MELROSE®, and RAVEN®

Raindrop and feather each oil on spine, as in Step 4 (Oregano).

Finger circles (after all three oils are applied).

Apply Zodiac Platonic 3rd (Om and Zodiac Platonic Earth forks) wherever muscle knots are found. Apply the Zodiac Platonic 3rd to the bank of muscles next to the spine, one side at a time. Walk up this band with the forks, moving about 2-3" each time, with Om closer to the feet and Zodiac Platonic Earth closer to the head. When completed, apply Om at the bottom of the band and Zodiac Platonic Earth at the top of the band.

6. MYRTLE

Sprinkle (6" above) from sacrum to atlas.

Feather stroke 3" straight up spine. Repeat with 6" then 12" strokes.

Thumb Vitaflex up spine.

Saw Maneuver up spine.

Stretch and Quiver up spine.

Apply the Full Sidereal Moon Major 6th (Om and Full Sidereal Moon forks) on the Huato Jiaji points up the spine from sacrum to base of skull, alternating the Full Sidereal Moon and Om forks on either side of the spine up to the atlas, then hold both forks at the crown of the head, GV-20.

7. ORTHO EASE®

Apply to entire back, followed by large circles with palms.

Palm Slide up & down the back. Apply more Ortho Ease® if needed.

Sound the High Jupiter 4th (High Om and High Jupiter forks) and move in a DN-8 figure over the client, from feet to crown, then back down off the feet.

8. VALOR®

Sprinkle (6" above) from sacrum to atlas.

Feather stroke 3" straight up spine. Repeat with 6" then 12" strokes.

Arched feather stroke 3" straight up spine. Repeat with 6" then 12" strokes.

Feather with full length strokes up and out, off the shoulders.

Sound the High New Synodic Moon 5th (High Om and High New Synodic Moon forks) and move in a DN-8 figure over the client, from feet to crown, then down off the feet.

9. RAVENSARA

Raindrop (6" above) 1-2 drops from sacrum to atlas. Feather as with Valor.

10. WARM COMPRESS

Apply hot compress; cool compress for MS clients.

Sound the High Full Sidereal Moon Major 6th (High Om and High Full Sidereal Moon forks), move in a DN-8 figure over the client from feet to crown, then down off the feet.

Apply the Om Octave (Om and Low Om forks) to the sole of each foot at KI-1 (Gushing Spring).

11 & 12   EVALUATE AND GIVE WATER

LUNG VRT:
Essential Oils

All of the Systems-specific Vibrational Raindrop Technique protocol use Valor, oregano and thyme as the core three oils to open and close Vibrational Raindrop Technique (EDOR, 4th Ed, page 299). Basil, marjoram, wintergreen, cypress and peppermint are replaced with oils more specific to the body system being treated. Details about the specific oils used to focus on the Lung system are included below.

RAVENSARA *(Ravensara aromatica)*

Family: Lamiaceae (mint family); antimicrobial and supporting to the nerves and respiratory system, called "the oil that heals" by the people of Madagascar. Contains 48-61% oxides, 16-32% monoterpenes. Ravensara is neutral and has an affinity to the Lung and Liver meridians. It can be used to Clear Wind Heat and Lung Heat with symptoms of fever, cough and wheezing. It can also be used for Lung Wind Cold with chest congestion and pain. Very pungent and dispersing, a strongly anti-viral essential oil.

MELROSE®

(Contains melaleuca, naouli, rosemary and clove); a strong topical antiseptic that cleans and disinfects cuts, scrapes, burns, rashes, and bruised tissue. Helps regenerate damaged tissue and reduce inflammation.

EUCALYPTUS RADIATA *(Eucalyptus radiata)*

Family: Myrtaceae (myrtle); antibacterial, antiviral, expectorant, used in respiratory and sinus infections; fights Herpes simplex when combined with bergamot. Contains 61-77% oxides, 13- 24% monoterpenes.

Warming with an affinity to the Lung and Stomach meridians, Eucalyptus Radiata is useful to treat Wind Cold with chills and fever, body aches, headaches and pain. It can be applied directly to the chest for Hot Phlegm and will expel Damp Phlegm.

MYRTLE *(Myrtus communis)*

Family: Myrtaceae (myrtle); normalizes hormonal imbalances, thyroid problems, prostate problems, and muscle spasms. Contains 31- 48% oxides, 30-45% monoterpenes.

Dry and cool, Myrtle clears Lung Heat and astringes leakage of qi and Blood such as sweating, bleeding, diarrhea, and hemorrhoids. It is calming as a nervine.

RAVEN®

(Contains ravensara, eucalyptus radiata, peppermint, wintergreen, and lemon); indicated for respiratory disease and infections such as tuberculosis, influenza and pneumonia; highly antiviral and antiseptic.

LUNG VRT:
Tuning Fork Intervals

Major Sixth, 3:5

Om/Full Sidereal Moon — Optimistic, less emotional than the Major 3rd; builds energy, brings a feeling of fullness, unveiling, and purification; the ultimate expression of Yin. Can bring a sense of magic and fulfillment; is rhythmic with a pull towards healing that allows one's potential to manifest. Known as the Golden Section, Divine Proportion, or Golden Mean. This interval builds yin energy, which moistens, consolidates and cools the body. It is especially effective for lung dryness that may come from smoking or emphysema.

Fifth, 2:3

High Om/High New Synodic Moon — calming, relaxing, and opening. The New Moon 5th is dispersive for emotional issues, while the Earth Day 5th is better suited to gather and strengthen energy. This interval opens, releases and dispels the stagnant energy that has accumulated during the Raindrop session, and is especially useful for asthma and lung congestion.

MACROCOSM: Planetary Frequencies and Vibrational Raindrop Technique (PLVRT)

Combining these sacred frequencies with the healing properties of essential oils, and applying them to ancient Chinese acupuncture points brings together multiple healing modalities, each with its own powerful morphic field.

Planetary Mythology

How did the planets get certain qualities associated with them? Usually it is because they have been associated with one of the ancient Greek/Roman gods or goddesses, and the associations have "stuck" over the centuries. Until the 17th century, a physician was not considered competent unless he was able to interpret the patient's birth chart, as well as the influence of the Heavens during one's lifetime. The influence of the planets and stars is still considered a part of some forms of medicine, such as Ayurvedic.

Sun *126.22 Hz, B1, -8th octave*
Function: Solar Plexus/Heart, Self, masculine, warming, leadership, power, initiatory. Heart, arteries, back, spine, physical vitality.

Associations: As the energetic center of gravity which the earth and other planets circle around, the sun is also the physical center of our galaxy. The frequency is calculated from an imaginary planet circling around the center of the sun to the minus 8th octave. It is a quantum physics calculation, and represents the border between Yin and Yang, or two opposites. Because it originates from a higher dimension, it stands for the magical and the transcendental.

Mythology: Helios/Apollo is the Good Shepherd with protective powers and skills for medicine and music. Apollo is the father of Asclepius and the foster parent of Chiron, two of the greatest healers in Greek mythology. Because he killed Asclepius's mother, Coronis, with an arrow, Apollo is powerless to heal arrow wounds.

Earth Day (Sidereal) *194.71 Hz, G2, 24th octave*
Function: Youthful, generative, dynamic, vitalizing. Body as a whole.

Associations: This is the first cosmic tuning of our planet, and its greatest influence is on the physical body. Its orbital frequency is about 4 minutes shorter than the average calendar day.

Mythology: Rhea/Gaia/Demeter is the Great Mother Goddess of the earth, fertility goddess, eternal parent, nurturing and loving creator of all life.

Earth Year (Om) *136.10 Hz, C2#, 32nd octave*
Function: Mother, grounding, soothing, balancing. Body as a whole.

Associations: This tone is based on the rotation of the earth around the sun with an orbital frequency of 365.242 days, which causes the changing of the seasons. This is the second cosmic rhythm of our planet. As the frequency of the Earth Day influences the body, the frequency of the Earth Year influences the soul. According to Hans Cousto, this tone is the keynote of sitar and tambura music as well as bells and other instruments in India. OM corresponds to the "Amen" in Christian churches. Meditation to this tone is deeply relaxing and calming to the soul.

Mythology: Rhea/Gaia/Demeter is the Great Mother Goddess of the earth, fertility goddess, eternal parent, nurturing and loving creator of all life.

Zodiac Earth (Platonic Year) *172.06 Hz, F2/F, 48th octave*

Function: Wisdom, clarity of spirit, expansive. Body as a whole.

Associations: This tone is the 48th octave of the precession of the earth's axis, the journeying of the vernal equinox through 25,920 years. At this time the vernal equinox has entered into the sign of Aquarius, hence we are in the "Age of Aquarius." F is the tone of the spirit, and was the fundamental tone in ancient China. In some systems, the tone F belongs to the crown chakra, the central point at the top of the head located at GV-20.

Mythology: Rhea/Gaia/Demeter is the Great Mother Goddess of the earth, fertility goddess, eternal parent, nurturing and loving creator of all life.

New Moon (Synodic) *210.42 Hz, G2#, 29th octave*

Function: Movement, feelings, communication, opening, feminine energy, nature, nurture. Stomach, breasts, lymph system, bodily fluids, childbirth, digestion.

Associations: The synodic month is the middle period from one New Moon to the next, and the calendar month is derived from this month. At New Moon the sun is in conjunction with the moon (the same direction in the sky). The tone of the New Moon is very suitable for meditation music at occasions like New Moon rituals. This tones improves general communication. In therapy the tone of the New Moon is frequently used with disturbances of the endocrine and lymph system as well as disturbances of menstruation.

Mythology: Diana/Artemis, daughter of Zeus and Leto, sister to Apollo, goddess of nature, protector of children and childbirth, and guardian of wild animals and the forest.

Full Moon (Sidereal) *227.43 Hz, A2#, 29th octave*

Function: Completeness, feelings, fullness, bridging, building, feminine, nature, nurture. Stomach, breasts, lymph system, bodily fluids, childbirth, digestion.

Associations: The orbital frequency of one revolution of the moon around the earth as measured against the celestial sphere. The sidereal month is about two and a quarter days shorter than a synodic month. This is caused by the apparent course of the sun along the ecliptic. As the sun passes approximately one sign per month, the moon has to pass through 13 signs to "keep up with it". At full moon, when sun is in opposition to the moon, people are more expansive than at new moon.

Mythology: Diana/Artemis, daughter of Zeus and Leto, sister to Apollo, goddess of nature, protector of children and childbirth, and guardian of wild animals and the forest.

Mercury *141.27 Hz, C2#, 30th octave*

Function: the Mind, intellectual communication, reason, dexterity. Nervous system, memory, thyroid, respiratory system and lungs, coordination, hands. It activates the mind and the reasoning faculty to promote knowledge, communication and synthesis.

Associations: Mercury is the planet next to the sun with a rotation around the sun of about 88 days. According to tradition, Mercury is associated as the morning star of Gemini and evening star of Virgo constellations.

Mythology: Mercury/Hermes is the messenger to the gods and also guides the souls of the dead to the underworld. Son of Zeus and Maia, brother of Apollo, makes the first musical instrument, lyre, from a tortoise shell and intestines.

Venus *221.23 Hz, A2/A, 32nd octave*

Function: relationships, higher love energy, aspiration for harmony. Throat, parathyroid, skeleton, kidneys and urinary tract, internal reproductive organs, capillaries and veins.

Associations: Venus is the second inner planet of our solar system and its rotation around the sun lasts about 225 days. According to tradition, Venus is associated as morning star of Taurus and evening star of Libra constellations. It brings beauty, harmony, creativity and abundance.

Mythology: Venus/Aphrodite is the goddess of love and beauty, born from the foam of Uranus's severed genitals falling into the sea, and is married to Haephestus, the blacksmith god.

Mars *144.72 Hz, D2/D, 33rd octave*

Function: Strength of will and focused energy, passion, survival, courage, power. Muscles, red blood cells, iron, adrenals, inflammation.

Associations: Mars is the first outer planet and has a rotation time of a little less than 2 years. Mars symbolizes the male focused energy, will and ability for achievement.

Mythology: Mars/Ares, known as the god of war, son of Zeus and Hera, lover of Venus/Aphrodite (his sister), ferocious in battle.

Jupiter *183.58 Hz, F2#, 36th octave*

Function: Expansion, evolution, creative power and continuous construction, philosophical and material creativity, joviality, generosity. Liver, glycogen, pancreas, insulin, hips/thighs, cellular growth and tumors.

Associations: Jupiter has a rotation time of a little less than 12 years. Jupiter is the largest of all planets and is situated in the middle of the known planets.

Mythology: Jupiter/Zeus, supreme god of the Olympian pantheon, god of light and sky, married to Hera. He escaped destruction by his father, Saturn/Kronos, and was reared far away from him. When Jupiter returns home, he forces his father to regurgitate his other offspring, and the siblings achieve rulership over the Titans.

Saturn *147.85 Hz, D2/D, 37th octave*

Function: Discipline, stability, patience, structure, limitation, protection, concentration, becoming conscious, karmic connections. Bones, cartilage, joints, knees, teeth, skin, ears.

Associations: Saturn is the last planet that can be seen with the naked eye. Its rotation time lasts about 29 years.

Mythology: Kronos/Saturn, the son of Uranus and Gaia, became the ruler over the physical universe when he castrated his father, Uranus (sky), in defense of his mother, Gaia (earth). Thus began a mythical Golden Age.

Uranus *207.36 Hz, G2#, 39th octave*

Function: Change, power of surprise and renewal, originality, electricity, revolution. Nervous conditions, lower legs/ankles/calves, pineal gland, electrical flow in the body.

Associations: Uranus is the first planet that cannot be seen with bare eyes. Its time of rotation lasts about 84 years. Uranus is generally associated with Aquarius in the zodiac. It was discovered in 1781. The planet Uranus is associated with the principle of falling and rising.

Mythology: Uranus is the Sky God with no Roman counterpart, married to Gaia, the Earth Goddess. Afraid of his children, he forbids Gaia to give birth to any more of them, though she is pregnant with many unborn children. Their son, Kronos, helps Gaia by castrating Uranus and throwing his genitals into the sea where they are the catalyst for the birth of Aphrodite.

Neptune *211.44 Hz, G2#, 40th octave*

Function: Transcendence, creativity, bliss, intuition, dream experience. Feet, thalamus, spinal cord and CSF, pineal, body water and mucus, edema, magnetic flow in the body, autoimmunity, right brain, appendix.

Associations: Neptune's rotation time lasts about 160 years, which is about two times the rotation time of Uranus. Looked at harmonically, Neptune is an octave lower than Uranus. Its tone is almost an octave analog that is equal to the New Moon. Neptune was discovered in 1846.

Mythology: Neptune/Poseidon, ruler of the sea, brother of Zeus/Jupiter and married to Hera/Juno. Swallowed by his father, Kronus, he was released by an emetic and is associated with the seas, oceans, lakes and earthquakes.

Pluto *140.25 Hz, C2#, 40th octave*

Function: Transformation, growth and transcendence through conflict, transmutation, shadow, death and resurrection. External reproductive organs, colon.

Associations: Pluto is known as the farthest planet from the Earth and was discovered in 1930. The time of rotation lasts about 250 years. Pluto is harmonically tuned to the New Moon and Neptune, with whom it has an exact quint-quint relation. Pluto is about 40 times farther away from the earth as the sun and a little smaller than the Earth's Moon.

Mythology: Pluto/Hades, ruler of the Underworld, brother of Zeus/Jupiter and married to Persephone (daughter of Gaia/Demeter). Hades tricks Persephone and abducts her to his realm, making her Queen of the Underworld. Her mother grieves and the earth begins to die, moving into Winter. Demeter is eventually able to arrange for Persephone to return to her 6 months of the year, which correspond to Spring and Summer. Because of the six pomegranate seeds that Persephone ate with Hades, she must return to the Underworld for 6 months (Fall and Winter).

Chiron (Healer), *151.27 Hz. D2#*

Function: Initiation, Destiny, Self-sacrifice, Compassion, Non-traditional healing methods. Left brain/right brain synthesis, wounds, bleeding, body minerals.

Associations: Discovered in 1977, Chiron is considered a planetoid and classified as a centaur. Centaurs are bodies originally from the Kuiper Belt which have been deflected into the region of Uranus and Saturn. They have a dual comet/asteroid nature, and thus have been named after the legendary Greek half man, half horse beings.

Mythology: Chiron, the "Wounded Healer", is a well-known figure in Greek mythology in the roots of medicine. Trained by Diana/Artemis and her brother, Apollo/Helios, he is expert in the arts of healing and war. He was half-man, half horse, and lived high on a mountain, alone in a cave. His famous pupils included Hercules, Achilles, Jason, and the great physician Aesculapius. One day Hercules, while drunk, gets into a fight with the other centaurs. He accidently shoots a stray poisoned arrow into Chiron's leg. However, Chiron cannot die because he is immortal, so he can only continue to exist in agony. He is the Wounded Healer who cannot cure himself, but awaits release from a Higher Source. Ultimately, he is able to bestow his immortality upon Prometheus, who lives a life of punishment by Zeus because he stole fire for humanity. Prometheus is released from the rock to which he has been chained, and the vultures can no longer feed upon him. Prometheus, the representative of mankind, is allowed to live forever by the sacrifice of the Wounded Healer.

MICROCOSM: Sacred Solfeggio and Vibrational Raindrop Technique (SSVRT)

The Solfeggio hexachord (6-tone scale) was rediscovered by Dr. Joseph Puleo, a naturopathic physician, in 1974 as a result of several mystical experiences of "conversations" with Jesus. Through a vision, Dr. Puleo was led to explore Psalms 119 and the Pythagorean method of reducing numbers to a single digit. He was then directed to the Book of Numbers, Chapter 7, beginning with Verse 12, and found the six musical frequencies that are hidden in the verse numbers. These original frequencies in Hertz are 396, 417, 528, 639, 741, and 852. According to Dr. Puleo, they were handed down to Levitical priests from ancient times, and were encrypted in the verse numbers of the Bible for safekeeping.*

These frequencies are used by healers all over the world, and have become well-known through the work of David Hulse, DD.

The hymn Ut Queant Laxis has an important place in the history of music. It is the basis of the solfege system of notation Ut (Do), Re, Mi, Fa, Sol, La, (Ti). Each phrase reflects the syllable and note. The most famous of the Hymn's melodies is the one used by the St. Cecilia Schola Cantorum, which correctly has each part of the first four lines start on the note higher than the previous one. The words of the hymn are attributed to Paul the Deacon as a tribute to Zacharias, the father of John the Baptist. The music was created by Guido of Arizzo, who perfected the new system of notation at that time, assisting singers to learn chants more easily. What exactly was the music used to sing the original solfeggio scale? This is not known because of the different tuning systems used throughout history. The original Solfeggio frequencies were supposedly part of this ancient chant to St. John the Baptist, which was lost several centuries ago.

Original hymn to John the Baptist reads as follows:
> UT queant laxis REsonare fibris
> MIra gestorum FAmuli tuorum
> SOLve pollute LAbii reatum
> Sancte Iohannes

Which translates into:
> *So that these your servants can, with all their voice, sing your wonderful feats, clean the blemish of our spotted lips, O Saint John!*

These frequencies have been made into tuning forks in 4 octaves, and can be used in Vibrational Raindrop Technique/VRT in many versions, which are outlined in this book.

Read more of Dr. Puleo's story in Healing Codes for the Biological Apocalypse by Leonard Horowitz and Joseph Puleo.

UT QUEANT LAXIS (HYMN TO ST. JOHN THE BAPTIST)

Guido of Arezzo
(circa 991-1033)

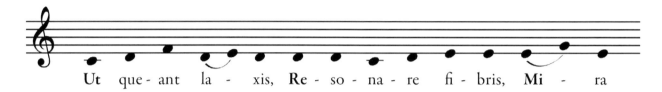

Ut que-ant la - xis, Re - so - na - re fi - bris, Mi - ra

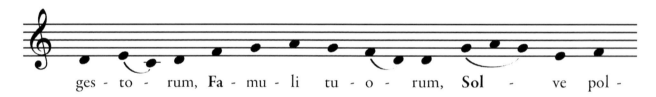

ges - to - rum, Fa - mu - li tu - o - rum, Sol - ve pol -

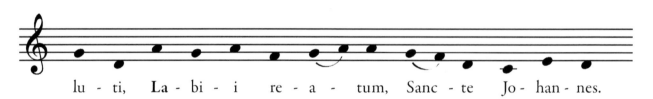

lu - ti, La - bi - i re - a - tum, Sanc - te Jo - han - nes.

Translation:

So that your servants may, with loosened voices, resound the wonders
of your deeds, clean the guilt from our stained lips, O Saint John.

ORIGIN OF THE
SACRED SOLFEGGIO FREQUENCIES

Through a vision from an angel, Dr. Joseph Puleo, a naturopathic doctor, was led to explore Psalms 119 and the Pythagorean method of reducing numbers to a single digit. The angel showed him the math that can be contained within language as well as the Pythagorean method of reducing numbers to a single digit.

He was then directed by Jesus/Jeshua to the book of Numbers, Chapter 7, Verses 12-83. He noticed that the verses had a repeating section of six verses that differed only in the day, the name of the offering person, and the tribe he came from. For instance, the first section of Verses 12-17, goes like this:

> ¹² And he that offered his offering the **first day was Nahshon the son of Amminadab**, of the tribe of **Judah**:
> ¹³ And his offering was one silver charger, the weight thereof was an hundred and thirty shekels, one silver bowl of seventy shekels, after the shekel of the sanctuary; both of them were full of fine flour mingled with oil for a meat offering:
> ¹⁴ One spoon of ten shekels of gold, full of incense:
> ¹⁵ One young bullock, one ram, one lamb of the first year, for a burnt offering:
> ¹⁶ One kid of the goats for a sin offering:
> ¹⁷ And for a sacrifice of peace offerings, two oxen, five rams, five he goats, five lambs of the first year: this was the offering of **Nahshon the son of Amminadab.**

The words in bold are the only items that will change in the next five sections through Verse 83. If you reduce the number of each verse to a single digit, then Verse 12 becomes a 3, Verse 13 becomes a 4, Verse 14 becomes a 5, and so on. So you have the first digits of your Sacred Solfeggio frequencies: 3, 4, 5, 6, 7, and 8.

The next set of numbers are found in the next section of Numbers, in Verses 18–23. Using the same process, you find the middle number in the Sacred Solfeggio frequencies: 9, 1, 2, 3, 4, and 5.

And the final set of numbers are found in the next section, Numbers: 24-29. Using the same Pythagorean process of reduction, the 3rd and final digit in the frequency code is 6, 7, 8, 9, 1, and 2. Put them all together and you have 396, 417, 528, 639, 741, and 852. Here's another way to break it down:

Verse 12 is 1+2 = 3
Verse 18 is 1+8 = 9
Verse 24 is 2+4 = 6
396 is the first frequency of UT
Verse 13 is 1+3 = 4
Verse 19 is 1+9 = 10 = 1
Verse 25 is 2+5 = 7
417 is the second frequency of RE
Verse 14 is 1+4 = 5
Verse 20 is 2+0 = 2
Verse 26 is 2+6 = 8
528 is the third frequency of MI
Verse 15 is 1+5 = 6
Verse 21 is 2+1 = 3
Verse 27 is 2+7 = 9
639 is the fourth frequency of FA
Verse 16 is 1+6 = 7
Verse 22 is 2+2 = 4
Verse 28 is 2+8 = 10 = 1
741 is the fifth frequency of SOL
Verse 17 is 1+7 = 8
Verse 23 is 2+3 = 5
Verse 29 is 2+9 = 11 = 2
852 is the sixth frequency of LA

The seventh tone and frequency is 963, and became SI for Sancte Iohannes, and then eventually TI. DO replaced UT because of its more open sound. The lower two frequencies were mathematically calculated in the same fashion with 174 (Soul Star) and 258 (Earth Star) as the result. All together you now have nine frequencies in the Sacred Solfeggio scale.

7 AND 12: A SACRED MARRIAGE

Is there any significance to the numbers 7 and 12, since they are where the Sacred Solfeggio frequencies encoding was found (chapter 7, verses 12+)? 7 and 12 have been called the "Supreme Numerical Marriage" because they bring together body (12) and soul (7). Juxtaposed against one another, they are the two great opposites in nature. The body is alive because of the soul, yet the soul needs the body for creation on this material plane.

The number 12 is the number of Universal Order. It is masculine and represents Light and the universal order in the heavenly city. It is seen in the chromatic scale of 12 tones, the 12 tribes/ nations, the 12 signs of the zodiac, 12 apostles, 12 gemstones of the breastplate, and much more. The geometry of 12 is beautifully proportioned, and easily drawn with a compass.

The number 7 is the number of the World Soul and mystery. It is feminine and represents Sound and the primordial, elemental world. It is not possible to divide a circle into seven exact portions, though one can get as close as 1/1000th. It is seen in the 7 churches, 7 golden candlesticks, 7 angels, 7 spirits of God, 7 kings, crowns, mountains, thunders, plagues, a Beast with 7 horns, a 7-headed dragon in Revelations.

According to John Mitchell in How The World Is Made, "In early classical societies these two opposites were ingeniously combined. A council of 12 elders decided the affairs of state, but every decision they took was referred to the state oracle, typically conducted by seven sibyls. If the oracle women foresaw trouble through any of the elders' decisions, they could veto it. In this way the interests of Twelve and Seven were happily balanced, following the old principle—man proposes, woman decides…

"In cosmologically ordered societies, in the traditional world plan they imitate, and in geometry itself, Seven and Twelve are bound together in a truly wonderful manner, completing through their union the image of creation that is the object of the Creator's quest."

JOHN THE BAPTIST

Known as the "voice crying in the wilderness", John the Baptist was called the greatest of all prophets, the Elijah who would precede the Messiah. John is *"the Elijah who is to come. Let anyone with ears listen!"* (Matthew 11:14). John foretold the coming of Christ, describing Him as one who would baptize with the "Holy Ghost and with fire."

He was born to the barren Elizabeth and her husband, Zacharias, a temple priest. Elizabeth was descended from the tribe of Levi (Luke 1:5) and was also related to Mary (Luke 1:36). Both Elizabeth and Zacharias were elderly, and John's birth had been foretold by the angel Gabriel. Because of their old age and the appearance of an angel, they considered her pregnancy a miracle. The angel Gabriel appeared to Zacharias while he was burning incense in the temple, and said to him, *"Do not be afraid, Zacharias, for your prayer is heard; and your wife Elizabeth will bear you a son, and you shall call his name John"* (Luke 1:13). The angel Gabriel assured Zacharias that his son would have a blessed mission in life. *"And you will have joy and gladness, and many will rejoice at his birth. For he will be great in the sight of the Lord, and shall drink neither wine nor strong drink. He will also be filled with the Holy Spirit, even from his mother's womb. And he will turn many of the children of Israel to the Lord their God. He will also go before Him in the spirit and power of Elijah, 'to turn the hearts of the fathers to the children,' (Malachi 4:6) and the disobedient to the wisdom of the just, to make ready a people prepared for the Lord"* (Luke 1:14-17).

Zacharias was stunned at the words and appearance of the angel, and expressed doubt. And Gabriel told him, *"you will be mute and not able to speak until the day these things take place, because you did not believe*

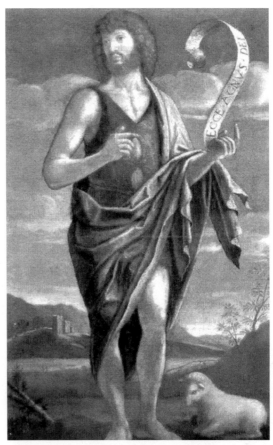

John the Baptist, courtesy Wikimedia Commons.

my words which will be fulfilled in their own time" (Luke 1:20).

When Zacharias left the temple to go to the people, he was unable to speak, just as Gabriel had foretold. He remained mute during the entire time of Elizabeth's pregnancy. When the day came for John's circumcision and naming, eight days after his birth, Elizabeth said that the child should be called John. No one accepted this name since she had no relatives with this name, and they asked Zacharias what the child should be named. *"And he asked for a writing tablet, and wrote, saying, 'His name is John.' . . . Immediately his mouth was opened and his tongue loosed, and he spoke, praising God"* (Luke 1:63-64).

Zacharias went on to speak a great prophesy about John and the guidance he would give his people and that he would prepare the way for the Lord (Luke 1:68-79). This is known as the Song of Zacharias or the Benedictus, and is a canticle sung at Lauds at daybreak.

During Elizabeth's pregnancy with John, her cousin Mary visited her. Mary had also received a visit from the angel Gabriel, who informed her that Elizabeth was six months' pregnant, and that Mary herself would bear a Son of God.

"And Mary arose in those days, and went into the hill country with haste, into a city of Judah; And entered into the house of Zacharias, and saluted Elisabeth. And it came to pass, that, when Elisabeth heard the salutation of Mary, the babe leaped in her womb; and Elisabeth was filled with the Holy Ghost: And she spake out with a loud voice, and said, Blessed art thou among women, and blessed is the fruit of thy womb. And whence is this to me, that the mother of my Lord should come to me? For, lo, as soon as the voice of thy salutation sounded in mine ears, the babe leaped in my womb for joy. And blessed is she that believed: for there shall be a performance of those things which were told her from the Lord."
(Luke 1:39-45).

Mary then spoke a joyful song (known as the Magnificat and sung at Vespers at sundown), stayed with Elizabeth for three months, then returned home. According to legend (Book of James, one of the Lost Books of the Bible), Zacharias and Elizabeth learned that Herod was seeking and slaying the children who were under two years old. Elizabeth took her 18-month-old infant son, John, *"up into the hillcountry and looked about her where she should hide him: and there was no hiding-place. And*

Elizabeth groaned and said with a loud voice: 'O mountain of God, receive thou a mother with a child.' For Elizabeth was not able to go up. And immediately the mountain clave asunder and took her in. And there was a light shining always for them: for an angel of the Lord was with them, keeping watch over them" (James 22:3).

Forty days later, Elizabeth died in the wilderness, and an angel took care of John the Baptist as he grew up in the desert, growing stronger in spirit all the time. "And the child grew, and waxed strong in spirit, and was in the deserts till the day of his shewing unto Israel"
(Luke 1:80).

Herod sent officers to Zacharias, demanding to know where his son was, but Zacharias denied any knowledge of John's whereabouts. Accordingly, he was brutally slain in the court of the temple, and his body could not be found; only his blood, hardened like stone.

John the Baptist lived an ascetic life in the desert with locusts and honey as his only food, and was said to have worn animal skins. "*Now John wore clothing of camel's hair with a leather belt around his waist, and his food was locusts and wild honey"* (Matthew 3:4). John has been called the Elijah who would precede the Messiah, and his description is reminiscent of Elijah, who was *"a hairy man, with a leather belt around his waist"* (II Kings 8). Priests and Levites from Jerusalem also asked John whether he was Elijah (John 1:20-21).

John began preaching in the wilderness of southern Judea around 27 AD, where there was a narrow band of green foliage, cane, tamarisk, brush and oleander. He baptized his followers in the River Jordan. He told his followers that they should repent because the kingdom of heaven was at hand. *"And so John came, baptizing in the desert region and preaching a baptism of repentance for the forgiveness of sins."* (Mark 1:4)

Baptism (Greek *baptizein*, "to immerse") was a well-known Jewish ritual that was practiced for several reasons, but repentance was one of the most common. One might also be baptized when converting to Judaism or when being initiated into ministry as a rabbi. His cousin, Jesus, was baptized by him as well *"in the fifteenth year of the reign of Emperor Tiberius, when Pontius Pilate was governor of Judea, and Herod was ruler of Galilee."* (Luke 3:1) This was about 28 A.D. since Tiberius became emperor in 14 AD, and Pontius Pilate became Roman Prefect in Judea in 26 AD.

At first John resisted Jesus's request to be baptized, saying, *"I need to be baptized by you, and (yet) you come to me?"* And Jesus answered him, *"Let it be so now; for it is proper for us in this way to fulfill all righteousness"* (Matthew 3:14-15). It was during this baptism that Jesus was informed of his mission as he emerged from the water. *"He saw the heavens torn apart and the Spirit descending like a dove on Him. And a voice came from heaven, 'You are my Son, the beloved; with you I am well pleased'"* (Mark 1:10-11). This verse is also seen in Matthew 3:16-17. In Luke 3:22 the dove is a physical manifestation of the Holy Ghost which was witnessed by all, and in John 1:32 only the Baptist was witness along with Jesus. The vision of the dove symbolizes the Spirit of the Lord anointing Jesus for His ministry as the Anointed One and Messiah. Again this is reminiscent of Isaiah's anointment by the Lord (Isaiah 61:1). Jesus quotes this very verse when he describes the beginning of His ministry (Luke 4:18).

Josephus, a Jewish scholar (37- c.100 AD), described John the Baptist as "a good man, who exhorted the Jews to exercise virtue, both in terms of righteousness toward one another and piety toward God, and so come to baptism" and says that the "Baptizer" was well liked. In Luke, he is shown to use words that shock his audience, warning them to stop being complacent and urge them to repentance.

John made some enemies along the way, including Herod Antipas and his wife Herodias. John preached against Herod because he had married his brother's wife. John told Herod, "it is not lawful for you to have your brother's wife" (Mark 6:18). After a drunken party, Herod promised Herodias's daughter, Salome, anything she wanted: she demanded the head of John the Baptist. John was in Herod's prison at the time, and he was accordingly beheaded. His head was brought to Salome on a large platter. His body was collected and buried by his disciples.

John's Feast days are June 24 (nativity) and August 29 (beheading). He is the patron of baptism, monastic life, and epileptics. His symbol is the lamb, and he is often shown with a long, narrow cross.

Primary appearances in the Bible: Matthew 3-17; Mark 1-6; Luke 1-3, 9; John 1-5.

SONG OF ZACHARIAS (BENEDICTUS)
LUKE 1: 67–79

The Benedictus was the song of thanksgiving uttered by Zacharias at the birth of his son, John the Baptist:

67 And his father Zacharias was filled with the Holy Ghost, and prophesied, saying,
68 Blessed be the Lord God of Israel; for he hath visited and redeemed his people,
69 And hath raised up an horn of salvation for us in the house of his servant David;
70 As he spake by the mouth of his holy prophets, which have been since the world began:
71 That we should be saved from our enemies, and from the hand of all that hate us;
72 To perform the mercy promised to our fathers, and to remember his holy covenant;
73 The oath which he sware to our father Abraham,
74 That he would grant unto us, that we being delivered out of the hand of our enemies might serve him without fear,
75 In holiness and righteousness before him, all the days of our life.
76 And thou, child, shalt be called the prophet of the Highest: for thou shalt go before the face of the Lord to prepare his ways;
77 To give knowledge of salvation unto his people by the remission of their sins,
78 Through the tender mercy of our God; whereby the dayspring from on high hath visited us,
79 To give light to them that sit in darkness and in the shadow of death, to guide our feet into the way of peace. (KJV)

The Benedictus (Song of Zacharias) is one of the three "evangelical canticles" (Benedictus from Zacharias is sung at Lauds, Magnificat from Virgin Mary is sung at Vespers, and Nunc dimittis from Simeon is sung at Compline) that are given in the opening chapters of Luke. Each of these canticles (hymns usually taken from scripture) honors the mystery of incarnation. All three of these canticles are sung every day, unlike the other canticles from the Old Testament which are sung only weekly. They are also positioned in the service in a way to give them great prominence, requiring the singers and congregation to stand while they are sung.

The first part of the canticle (verses 68-75) is a song of thanksgiving for the Jewish nation that they would now be delivered from oppression by their enemies by the family of David as the fulfillment of God's oath to Abraham. This deliverance has a glorious goal, that they "might serve him without fear, In holiness and righteousness before him, all the days of our life."

Zacharias addresses his son, John, directly in the second part of the canticle (verses 76-78), praising his role as prophet to prepare the way for "the face of the Lord" and assist the people in redeeming their sins.

St. Benedict of Nursia is believed to have first introduced the use of this canticle in the services of the Roman Catholic Church. It is one of the canticles in the Anglican service of Morning Prayer/Matins according to the Book of Common Prayer. It may also be used as a canticle in the Lutheran service of Matins.

The canticle was originally written in Greek, in the Gospel of Luke, and is shown below translated into Latin, then into English for the Douay-Rheims Bible in the service of the Catholic Church, and finally in the Book of Common Prayer for the Anglican Church.

Greek

Εὐλογητὸς κύριος ὁ θεὸς τοῦ Ἰσραήλ,

ὅτι ἐπεσκέψατο καὶ ἐποίησεν λύτρωσιν τῷ λαῷ αὐτοῦ,

καὶ ἤγειρεν κέρας σωτηρίας ἡμῖν

ἐν οἴκῳ Δαυὶδ παιδὸς αὐτοῦ,

καθὼς ἐλάλησεν διὰ στόματος τῶν ἁγίων ἀπ' αἰῶνος προφητῶν αὐτοῦ,

σωτηρίαν ἐξ ἐχθρῶν ἡμῶν καὶ ἐκ χειρὸς πάντων τῶν μισούντων ἡμᾶς·

ποιῆσαι ἔλεος μετὰ τῶν πατέρων ἡμῶν

καὶ μνησθῆναι διαθήκης ἁγίας αὐτοῦ,

ὅρκον ὃν ὤμοσεν πρὸς Ἀβραὰμ τὸν πατέρα ἡμῶν,

τοῦ δοῦναι ἡμῖν

ἀφόβως ἐκ χειρὸς ἐχθρῶν ῥυσθέντας

λατρεύειν αὐτῷ ἐν ὁσιότητι

καὶ δικαιοσύνῃ ἐνώπιον αὐτοῦ πάσαις ταῖς ἡμέραις ἡμῶν.

Καὶ σὺ δέ, παιδίον, προφήτης ὑψίστου κληθήσῃ,

προπορεύσῃ γὰρ ἐνώπιον κυρίου ἑτοιμάσαι ὁδοὺς αὐτοῦ,

τοῦ δοῦναι γνῶσιν σωτηρίας τῷ λαῷ αὐτοῦ

ἐν ἀφέσει ἁμαρτιῶν αὐτῶν,

διὰ σπλάγχνα ἐλέους θεοῦ ἡμῶν,

ἐν οἷς ἐπισκέψεται ἡμᾶς ἀνατολὴ ἐξ ὕψους,

ἐπιφᾶναι τοῖς ἐν σκότει καὶ σκιᾷ θανάτου καθημένοις,

τοῦ κατευθῦναι τοὺς πόδας ἡμῶν εἰς ὁδὸν εἰρήνης.

Latin

Benedictus Dominus Deus Israel; quia visitavit et fecit redemptionem plebi suae

et erexit cornu salutis nobis, in domo David pueri sui,

sicut locutus est per os sanctorum, qui a saeculo sunt, prophetarum eius,

salutem ex inimicis nostris, et de manu omnium, qui oderunt nos;

ad faciendam misericordiam cum patribus nostris, et memorari testamenti sui sancti,

iusiurandum, quod iuravit ad Abraham patrem nostrum, daturum se nobis,

ut sine timore, de manu inimicorum liberati, serviamus illi

in sanctitate et iustitia coram ipso omnibus diebus nostris.

Et tu, puer, propheta Altissimi vocaberis: praeibis enim ante faciem Domini parare vias eius,

ad dandam scientiam salutis plebi eius in remissionem peccatorum eorum,

per viscera misericordiae Dei nostri, in quibus visitabit nos oriens ex alto,

illuminare his, qui in tenebris et in umbra mortis sedent, ad dirigendos pedes nostros in viam pacis.

From the Douay-Rheims Bible (1582)

Blessed be the Lord God of Israel; because he hath visited and wrought the redemption of His people:
And hath raised up an horn of salvation to us, in the house of David his servant:
As he spoke by the mouth of his holy prophets, who are from the beginning:
Salvation from our enemies, and from the hand of all that hate us:
To perform mercy to our fathers, and to remember his holy testament,
The oath, which he swore to Abraham our father, that he would grant to us,
That being delivered from the hand of our enemies, we may serve him without fear,
In holiness and justice before him, all our days.
And thou, child, shalt be called the prophet of the Highest: for thou shalt go before the face of the Lord to prepare his ways:
To give knowledge of salvation to his people, unto the remission of their sins:
Through the bowels of the mercy of our God, in which the Orient from on high hath visited us:
To enlighten them that sit in darkness, and in the shadow of death: to direct our feet into the way of peace.

From the Book of Common Prayer (1662)

Blessed be the Lord God of Israel: for he hath visited, and redeemed his people;
And hath raised up a mighty salvation for us: in the house of his servant David;
As he spoke by the mouth of his holy Prophets: which have been since the world began;
That we should be saved from our enemies: and from the hands of all that hate us;
To perform the mercy promised to our forefathers: and to remember his holy Covenant;
To perform the oath which he sware to our forefather Abraham: that he would give us;
That we being delivered out of the hands of our enemies: might serve him without fear;
In holiness and righteousness before him: all the days of our life.
And thou, Child, shalt be called the Prophet of the Highest: for thou shalt go before the face of the Lord to prepare his ways;
To give knowledge of salvation unto his people: for the remission of their sins,
Through the tender mercy of our God: whereby the day-spring from on high hath visited us;
To give light to them that sit in darkness, and in the shadow of death: and to guide our feet into the way of peace.

GUIDO D'AREZZO AND THE UT-RE-MI SOLMIZATION

Born in France around 995, Guido of Arezzo (also known as Guido Aretinas) served as a Benedictine monk and reportedly was a young music scholar of great talent. He was also a gifted teacher and is the inventor of modern musical notation that replaced neumatic notation.

While serving as the young head of the cathedral choir school in Arezzo, Guido developed innovative ways to instruct his choir. Keep in mind that music was learned by heart at that time; there were no music sheets or piano keyboard. There were only small signs called neumes written over the words of a text. These inflective marks would show the general shape of a melody but not the exact notes or the rhythm.

Guido would point to the four fingers of his left hand or the spaces in between when guiding his choir in rehearsal. He explained that the various points on his hand always made the same sound. Later, he put hand points onto written staves, again explaining that notes on the same line had the same tone.

Then he taught his students about rhythm and the metrical quality of chants. The choir learned about dactyls, spondees, iambics, pentameters and other forms of rhythm from ancient lyric poets. He also introduced a system of solmization; the solfegge, or Aretinian syllables ut, re, mi, fa, sol and la. These syllables were used as names for the six tones C, D, E, F, G and A, the hexachord. One day, he started assigning these letters to the sounds, and then assigned the sounds to a hymn, Ut Queant Laxis, in praise of John the Baptist.

The Micrologus de disciplina artis musicae (c. 1025), is the book written by Guido about his teaching system. It was an extremely effective method to learn music, and Guido's students were able to learn in days what usually took weeks to master. They sang with perfect pitch, and their cathedral was overflowing with worshippers who came to listen. And so Guido's fame spread.

The "Guidonian Hand" was used widely as a teaching tool. Parts of each finger were assigned a different note. Guido and his followers could teach singers their notes by pointing to different parts of the hand. In 1028, he demonstrated this and other innovative teaching methods to Pope John XIX.

The Hymn: Ut Queant Laxis

Guido connected his melody to the text of a famous hymn in honor of John the Baptist of which the first stanza is as follows:

Ut queant laxis resonare fibris
mira gestorum famuli tuorum,
solve polluti labii reatum,
Sancte Ioannes.
*So that your servants may sound forth
the wonders of your deeds with loosened hearts,
remove the guilt of our tainted lips,
Saint John.*

Since each half-line of the first three verses begins on a progressively higher note, Guido used the first syllable of each half-line (shown in bold) to generate the series **ut–re–mi–fa–so–la.** Ut was changed to the open syllable Do in 1600 in Italy, at the suggestion of the musicologue Giovanni Battista Doni, and SI (from the initials for Sancte Iohannes) was added to complete the diatonic scale. In Anglo-Saxon countries, SI was changed to TI by Sarah Glover in the nineteenth century so that every syllable might begin with a different letter. With Ut replaced by Do and with the addition of TI and a second Do to complete the octave, Guido's mnemonic forms the basis of the solfège or solmization system still in use today.

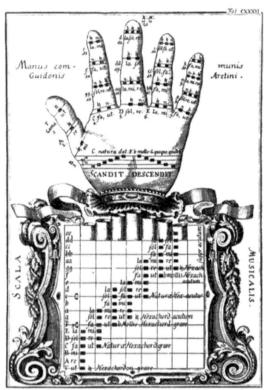

The Guidonian hand - Guido of Arezzo's device for showing the notes of the scale (Italian theorist, music teacher and Benedictine monk, b c.991-d after 1033). The dotted line shows the order in which the notes are to be read.

Where did the Melody arise?

We now know where the solfege syllables were created, and we know the probable origin of the words of the Hymn to John the Baptist. But where did the melody arise? The hymn known at Ut Queant Laxis can be heard performed by various chanters today, and it is a hauntingly beautiful yet simple melody. But it does not sound like the frequencies that we use in the Sacred Solfeggio tuning forks.

Many scholars believe that the melody in question was first used for Ut Queant Laxis and later transferred to Horace's Ode to Phyllis, but more recent opinion is that Horace's music was used by Guido. An enlightening and engaging account in support of this argument can be read in Horace's Odes and the Mystery of Do-Re-Mi by Stuart Lyons, former senior Classics scholar at King's College, Cambridge. He successfully weaves the argument that Guido indeed had a manuscript with this Ode to Phyllis that was complete with musical notes written over the words, which increased a note with each stanza. The Ode to Phyllis is written in Sapphic stanza, as is Ut Queant Laxis, so moving the melody from one to the other was simple.

Guido never revealed the source of the melody, no doubt because an Ode by Horace would not have been considered reverent. However, Horace died only a few years before both John the Baptist's and Jesus's births, so a melody from this era seems entirely appropriate.

This hymn itself is attributed to Paul the Deacon who was born into a noble Lombard family about 720. A Benedictine monk, he spent much of his life teaching and writing many works of history for the Duke of Benevento. But his great love was to write Latin verses, and when he retired to the great monastery of Monte Cassino, he wrote the hymn, Ut Queant Laxis. His many literary achievements attracted the attention of Charlemagne, with whom he was acquainted and to whom he dedicated one of his works. It is popularly thought that Paul wrote Ut Queant Laxis on the Holy Saturday when he was hoarse and feared he could not chant the Easter Proclamation. He was reminded of the loss of voice by Zacharias, the father of John the Baptist, and its subsequent restoration through faith.

HARMONICS

What is the difference between resonance and harmonics? Resonance occurs from without; harmonics occur from within. We respond to harmonics at a cellular level.

According to Wikipedia, "A harmonic of a wave is a component frequency of the signal that is an integer multiple of the fundamental frequency, i.e. if the fundamental frequency is f, the harmonics have frequencies 2f, 3f, 4f…" and so on. These relationships between members of the series remain constant, no matter what the Fundamental (f) is. A harmonic series can have any note as its fundamental, so there are many different harmonic series. But remember: the relationship between the frequencies of a harmonic series is always the same. The second harmonic always has exactly half the wavelength (and twice the frequency) of the fundamental; the third harmonic always has exactly a third of the wavelength (and so three times the frequency) of the fundamental, and so on.

Shown below is a chart of the harmonics if the Fundamental (f) = 136.10 (Om) that goes up to 7 times the Fundamental frequency. I've also shown the level at which the harmonic interval has its greatest effect

in terms of energetic anatomy. For instance, the 3rd Harmonic (2nd overtone of 136.10 Hz) is a Perfect 5th and affects the Lower Emotional Body. These harmonics grow increasingly faint as they rise, but the first six all repeat the pitches of what we know as the "major triad" (octave, 5th, 3rd) based on the Fundamental.

You will see that the interval of the Octave is unique; it is obtained by doubling or halving the rate of vibration. It is the "frame" for musical scales everywhere, and can be divided into many smaller intervals to make different scales. Usually it is divided into 7 intervals framed by 8 tones; hence the word "octave." When there are only the 8 tones, it is referred to as a diatonic octave; if it includes all 12 tones, it is called a chromatic octave.

These 7 intervals can be termed consonant or dissonant, according to the human response to the interval. In some ways, our responses are subjective and have changed over the centuries. In medieval times, the only pleasant sounding, consonant intervals were the octave, perfect 5th and perfect 4th. This has changed over time, and Thirds and Sixths are well-liked by many people today. Even Seconds and Sevenths are found appealing, some of the time by some of the people.

Frequency	Energy Body	Tone/Overtone	Harmonic	Harmonic Interval
1 • f = 136.1 Hz	Physical	FUNDAMENTAL TONE	1st	Fundamental
2 • f = 272.2 Hz	Etheric	1st overtone	2nd	1st Octave
3 • f = 408.29 Hz	Lower Emotional	2nd overtone	3rd	Perfect 5th
4 • f = 544.4 Hz	Heart	3rd overtone	4th	2nd Octave
5 • f = 680.5 Hz	Higher Emotional	4th overtone	5th	Major 3rd
6 • f = 816.6 Hz	Mental	5th overtone	6th	Perfect 5th
7 • f = 952.7 Hz	Spiritual	6th overtone	7th	Minor 7th

Third Force

But our response to musical intervals actually has objective physics behind it. When most vibrations of differing frequencies interact, some dissonance appears in the form of what is called a third vibration, or "third force." The octave, however, is totally consonant, as the interaction of the two tones that compose it make no third vibration, or force.

The next most consonant interval is the Fifth, commonly called the Perfect 5th, which produces a tiny amount of dissonance in the form of a third force.

Next is the Fourth, which produces slightly more third force.

As we move down the scale of dissonant intervals, the 12th interval from total consonance toward increasing dissonance is the Augmented 4th, or Tritone. It is so dissonant that at one point in the history of music, it was referred by the Church as the "devil's tone." It is the most unstable of intervals as a harmony and difficult to sing as melody, because acoustically its pitches have nothing in common; there is no reinforcement between them. Since Third Force is so dissonant, it is a vehicle to move Qi and assist the person to find their natural state of balance.

Here is the order of consonance to dissonance in a chromatic scale: Octave/Unison, Fifth, Fourth, Major 3rd, minor 3rd, Major 6th, minor 6th, Major 2nd, Major 7th, minor 2nd, minor 7th, Augmented 4th (tritone).

We have been primarily discussing Western music so far. In Eastern music, there is a monophonic system that uses only melodies, not intervals or chords. It has many microtones, which are intensely dissonant. It is thought that these notes operate on the Inner Octaves to affect the inner states of humans and animals.

REVIEW OF SCALES, INTERVALS, AND TONES

A note is a tone is a pitch. There are seven main pitches or tones in the diatonic musical scale (A through G) and these are the white keys on a piano. But there are 12 possible notes (12 half steps, each worth 100 cents) in an octave, which is called a chromatic scale. The extra 5 notes fall between the seven main tones, and are the black keys (sharps and flats) on a piano. Each pitch/key is the same interval away from the previous pitch/key. A sharp raises the natural note, and a flat lowers the note. In a tempered scale, C# is the same as Db, since the half step is always 100 cents. In a Just scale, there is a slight difference between a sharp and a flat. There are nine commas in the interval of a single tone from one note to the next, i.e., from C to D, from D to E, and so on. This is important if one needs to know that there is a difference between Db and C#, for instance. Db is 4 commas above C, while C# is 6 commas above C. The middle of the C to D interval is at 5 commas. An octave is the interval between one musical tone and another with half or double its frequency. All scales start on one note and end on that same note one octave higher.

We will often be referring to three major types of scales. Equal-tempered scale refers to 12-tone equal temperament with intervals corresponding to 100 cent multiples (e.g., 100, 200, 300, etc.). Just means 5-limit just intonation—a ratio of numbers with prime factors no higher than five. Pythagorean means 3-limit just intonation—a ratio of numbers with prime factors no higher than three. We are usually working in the Just Scale, though the other two scales are important to understand.

An **interval** is the distance between two notes, and the sound that results when these two tones are sounded at the same time. It is a point that results from the meeting of the two waves of two tones. Some intervals are naturally and traditionally pleasing ("consonant") such as the octave (2:1), fifths (3:2) and fourths (4:3). These consonant ratios were used to create architecture in the Ancient world, and the most beautiful temples of Athens, Rome and Egypt are based upon these proportions.

Of special interest in the Sacred Solfeggio scale are the intervals of the Fourth and Fifth:

The **4th interval** is also known by its Greek name, Diatesseron. According to the Oxford English Dictionary, Diatessaron (daɪəˈtɛsərən) means the interval of a fourth. However, that is considered an old and obsolete use. The more common meaning is "A harmony of the four Gospels." This is derived from the title of the earliest work of the kind, the 2nd century Εὐαγγέλιον διὰ τεσσάρων, i.e. 'gospel made up of four', of Tatian. More recent examples of the use of this meaning include:

> 1803 T. Thirlwall (title), Diatessaron; or the History of our Lord Jesus.
> 1805 R. Warner (title), The English Diatessaron; or the History of Christ, from the compounded Texts of the Four Evangelists.

So it seems especially appropriate that these Sacred Solfeggio frequencies have Perfect Fourths and nearly perfect Augmented Fourths contained within them.

A Perfect 4th in just intonation corresponds to a pitch ratio of 4:3, or about 498 cents, while in equal temperament a Perfect 4th is equal to five semitones, or 500 cents. Some well-known examples are the starting of the "Bridal Chorus" from Wagner's *Lohengrin* (*"Treulich geführt"*, the colloquially-titled "Here Comes the Bride"); the first two notes of the Christmas carol "Hark! The Herald Angels Sing"; and, for a descending perfect fourth, the second and third notes of "O Come All Ye Faithful".

Fabien Maman describes the Fourth interval as "Awakening and at the same time paralyzing… we begin to awaken from emotion. The fourth interval… is like awakening from a dream." According to John Beaulieu, the Fourth can be very grounding and stabilize hyper or obsessive thoughts. It "balances the fourth ventricle of the brain and releases opiate receptors in the fourth ventricle; down-regulates amygdala…"

An **Augmented 4th (Tritone)** has a pitch ratio of 45:32, 600 cents in equal temperament, and is an interval consisting of three whole tones (six semitones). In 1609, Douland (Ornith. Microl. 20) said, 'A Tritone doth exceed the Consonance of a Diatessaron.' In 1789 Burney (Hist. Mus. (ed. 2) III. vii. 344) said, 'The Tritonus, consisting of three tones, without the intervention of a semitone, is extremely difficult to sing.' Over the years, the Augmented 4th has been recognized as a difficult pitch to sing, and falls within that void in musical scales: between two notes which are separated from one another by a whole step.

Some modern examples include the theme opening Claude Debussy's *Prélude à l'après-midi d'un faune* that outlines a tritone (between C# and G), which has a hauntingly beautiful quality. George Harrison of the Beatles favored this interval, using it in the opening phrases of "The Inner Light", "Blue Jay Way" and "Within You Without You".

Fabien Maman says that the left and right sides of the brain are stimulated by the Augmented 4th, and that it is the sound heard with a Tibetan singing bowl. The tension of this interval is maintained until it finds resolution in the Perfect 5th interval.

While it was usually avoided in medieval ecclesiastical singing because of its dissonance, it was Guido of Arezzo who explicitly prohibited its use! In his hexachord system, B flat was introduced as a diatonic note (the fourth degree of the hexachord on F). From that time forward, it

was called the diabolus in musica ("the Devil in music"), regarded as far too unstable, and was rejected. The idea that singers were excommunicated or otherwise punished by the Church for invoking this interval are not likely true. Avoidance of the interval for musical reasons has a long history for good reasons. (Please see the section on Sacred Solfeggio Intervals for specifics on this issue.)

The **Perfect 5th interval** is associated with the nitrogen atom, according to Joachim Berendt, and stimulates nitric oxide release by an unknown mechanism (Beaulieu 2003). Beaulieu postulates that nitric oxide acts locally as a hormone as well as a neurotransmitter and is antibacterial and antiviral, enhances the immune system, balances the heart, pituitary gland and sphenoid bone, balances the autonomic nervous system, releases opiate and cannabinoid receptor sites in the brain's third ventricle. It enhances the mobility of joints, and can relieve depression.

Music exists in movement, starting from a specific point, moving through different notes or intervals to create tension, and releasing. Consonance and dissonance arise when two notes are sounded together, creating an interval which is either pleasing and relaxing (consonant) or unstable, energetic and full of movement (dissonant). These are not absolute definitions since the response to an interval is highly subjective and related to cultural background. In our modern Western world, we experience most intervals as relatively consonant and pleasing. But the 2nds and 7ths are the most dissonant and therefore full of tension. They can be used to generate a high state of energy and movement, and are critical for growth and evolution.

An interval's quality is determined by its relationship to the Fundamental tone within the system being used. Please see the section on Sacred Solfeggio intervals for more on this topic.

SACRED SOLFEGGIO CHART

	2 Octaves Lower	1 Octave Lower	Original Frequencies	1 Octave Higher		
NAME	LOW weighted	MID weighted	HIGH unweighted	ANGELIC unweighted	LATIN NAME & MEANING	CHAKRA
Soul	43.5 Hz (=3)	87 Hz (=6)	**174 Hz (=3)**	348 Hz (=6)	**Soul** Becomes Light Spirit into Matter	**Soul Star**
Earth	71.25 Hz (=6)	142.5 Hz (=3)	**285 Hz (=6)**	570 Hz(=3)	**Earth** Energy Fields, Unification with Gaia Grounding	**Earth Star**
UT	99 Hz (=9)	198 Hz (=9)	**396 Hz (=9)**	792 Hz (=9)	**UT queant laxis Emotional Release** Liberating Guilt and Fear	**Root**
RE	104.25 Hz (=3)	208.5 Hz (=6)	**417 Hz (=3)**	834 Hz (=6)	**REsonare fibris Transform** Undoing Situations and Facilitating Change	**Sacral**
MI	132 Hz (=6)	264 Hz (=3)	**528 Hz (=6)**	1056 Hz (=3)	**MIra gestorum Miracle DNA** Transformation and Miracles (DNA Repair)	**Solar Plexus**
FA	159.75 Hz (=9)	319.5 Hz (=9)	**639 Hz (=9)**	1278 Hz (=9)	**FAmuli tuorum** Connecting/Relationships	**Heart**
SOL	185.25 Hz (=3)	370.5 Hz (=6)	**741 Hz (=3)**	1482 Hz (=6)	**SOLve polluti** Awakening Intuition	**Throat**
LA	213 Hz (=6)	426 Hz (=3)	**852 Hz (=6)**	1704 Hz (=3)	**LAbii reatum** Returning to Spiritual Order	**3rd Eye**
TI	240.75 Hz (=9)	481.5 Hz (=9)	**963 Hz (=9)**	1926 Hz (=9)	**Sancte Ioannes** Conscious Disciplined Connection to Spirit Matter into Spirit	**Crown**

MEANINGS OF THE SACRED SOLFEGGIO FREQUENCIES

Soul Star – 43 Hz, 87 Hz, 174 Hz, 348 Hz
Soul becomes Light, reducing pain and blockages

The Soul Star frequency releases energy blockages, which is the key to reducing pain according to the Chinese medicine world. Imagine every nerve, blood vessel, muscle, organ, etc., in your body being bathed in its own freely moving energy! The journey begins as spirt as turned into matter.

Earth Star – 71.25 Hz, 142.5 Hz, 285 Hz, 570 Hz
Balance with earth's energy fields, unifying with Gaia

As the electromagnetic energy begins to move more freely, the body is able to heal itself, and tissues may return to its original form. This frequency vibrates on deep energy field levels to rejuvenate your body at one of the deepest levels and ground spiritual energy.

UT – 99 Hz, 198 Hz, 396 Hz, 792 Hz
Turning grief into joy, liberating guilt & fear

This tone is said to liberate and cleanse the emotions of guilt and fear, which often represent basic obstacles to joy and returning to our original perfection. Joy can come out of released negative emotions. The UT frequency searches out hidden blockages and subconscious negative beliefs that are linked to your present situation, whether it is physical, emotional, mental and/or spiritual. It is a preparatory tone to prepare the body on all levels to receive the next six tones.

It is especially useful when used in combination with phenolic compounds in essential oils, which share the qualities of acting as protective agents, inhibitors and natural defenders against invading organisms. Phenylpropanoids are phenols with one isoprene unit attached and come in many varieties with a molecular weight of 136 amu. Examples frequently used in VRT would be oregano, basil, and thyme to clean the receptor sites.

RE – 104.25 Hz, 208.5 Hz, 417 Hz, 834 Hz
Undoing situations and facilitating change

In order to change, we need to have enough energy to undertake the task. The RE frequency provides the energy to cleanse traumatic experiences and clear destructive influences of past events out of our cellular memory.

Sesquiterpene compounds in essential oils resonate with the high energy necessary to cleanse the unnecessary "garbage" from the cellular experiences and memories. Examples include cedarwood, vetiver, spikenard, sandalwood, myrrh and thousands more. Sesquiterpenes are made of three isoprene units (formula C_5H_8 and 68 amu) with a formula of $C_{15}H_{24}$ and a molecular weight of 204 amu.

MI – 132 Hz, 264 Hz, 528 Hz, 1056 Hz
Transformation and miracles (DNA repair)

The MI frequency is said to bring transformation and miracles into your life, to return human DNA to its "original, perfect state." The process of DNA repair is followed by the free flow of electromagnetic energy/Qi. This increases our clarity of mind, awakened or activated creativity, and increased life energy. When a negative feeling is released (UT) and removed (RE) from our DNA, we prepare the way for the possibility of every problem (physical, mental, emotional, and spiritual) and inappropriate behavior based on old stuck emotions to quickly disappear from our lives.

The best and most abundant essential oils would be ones with monoterpene compounds such as frankincense, angelica, hyssop, galbanum, peppermint and many, many more! Monoterpenes are compounds composed of two isoprene units (formula $C5H8$ and 68 amu) which have the general formula $C10H16$ with a molecular weight of 136 amu.

FA – 159.75 Hz, 319.5 Hz, 639 Hz, 1278 Hz
Re-connecting and balancing, relationships

The FA tone can be used to seek out limitations that seem to be imposed upon us. It enables the creation of a harmonious community and harmonious interpersonal relationships because it enhances communication, understanding, tolerance and love. It is the middle of the octave, and higher energies with greater help begin to enter the process. FA can be used for relationship problems – those in family, between partners, friends or social relationships. At a cellular process level, this frequency can be used to encourage the cell to communicate with its environment.

SOL – 185.25 Hz, 370.5 Hz, 741 Hz, 1482 Hz
The awakening of consciousness, solving problems, expressions/solutions

It cleans the cellular energetic matrix ("Solve polluti") from energetic toxins and various electromagnetic radiations. This sound frequency can be used for solving problems of any nature, and increase one's power of self-expression, as we are more receptive to higher truths and principles. It is a tone to loosen, release, unbind, untie, open and free expression and communication.

LA – 213 Hz, 426 Hz, 852 Hz, 1704 Hz
Awakening intuition, returning to spiritual order

LA assists in allowing clarity of vision, both the physically visible as well as the energetically visible. It unveils the illusions in life ("maya") and hidden agendas of people, places and things. This is also a good tone to open the vocal cords and "release the lips." Our lives acquire a quality of effortlessness and are without any struggle because we have surrendered to the Divine Love which resonates in this frequency.

TI – 240.75 Hz, 481.5 Hz, 963 Hz, 1926 Hz

Conscious disciplined connection to spirit

Radical transformation and spiritual awakening are the highlight with this frequency, and the emotion is one of gratefulness. It is connected with the Light and all-embracing Spirit, and will assist one to become a model of enlightened engagement with the world in which we live. There is a higher power within the potential of this frequency in which we must learn to trust. This will enable one to experience Oneness—our true nature, as matter returns to spirit.

LAW OF THE OCTAVE, SOLFEGGIO HEXACHORD SCALE AND THREE EXTRA TONES

The Sacred Solfeggio scale rediscovered by Dr. Joseph Puleo is a hexachord with 6 tones. These original tones are 396 Hz, 417 Hz, 528 Hz, 639 Hz, 741 Hz and 852 Hz. Additional frequencies have been calculated using the pattern established by the six original tones. There are two frequencies which have been calculated below the 396 (174 Hz and 285 Hz) and there is one frequency above the 852 which we use (963 Hz).

Following the Law of the Octave, additional frequencies can be calculated at various octaves. The use of these other octaves enables the application of various weighted and unweighted tuning forks, allowing one to access each octave's different energy fields at the appropriate levels.

The Law of the Octave was first described in 1865 by John Newlands, an English chemist, who noticed that the 56 elements known at that time could be grouped into divisions with similar chemical properties, and that the different members had atomic numbers which varied by 8 (sodium/Na = 11, potassium/K = 19 and so on). It reminded him of the Pythagorean musical scale, and he called it the "Law of the Octave." The Russian chemist Mendeleyev created the Periodic Table of the Elements in the 1870s, "an octave of hauntingly Pythagorean harmony" according to Robert Anton Wilson. His concept was ridiculed until the ideas of electron valence were postulated in the early 1900s.

More recently, in 1978 Hans Cousto, a Swiss mathematician and musicologist, discovered the natural law of the "Cosmic Octave" as the link between different kinds of periodically occurring natural phenomena, such as the orbit of the planets, the weather, colors, rhythms and tones. "The law of the octave is this principle where mathematics and music equally partake. This law makes it possible to combine astronomical and musical formulas," Cousto says. In music, octaves are considered to have the same tone that is proportionally higher or lower. For instance, Middle C (C4 on a piano equal to 261.626 Hz) has the same tone as C1, C2, C3, C5 and so on. And the frequencies of these other "C"s are multiples of 2 in relation to each other. If Middle C (C4) is 261.626 Hz, then Bass C (C3) is half that (130.813 Hz), Low C (C2) is half of C3 (65.406 Hz), and Tenor C (C5) is double C4 (523.251 Hz). Harmonically, octaves have the most consonant sound of all: there is virtually no "third force" frequency or sound when playing an octave. You can test this out by playing two tuning forks together that are an octave apart. There should be no "wobble" or extra beats to the sound that you hear.

PERIODIC TABLE OF THE ELEMENTS

LIST OF JUST SCALE INTERVALS USED IN SACRED SOLFEGGIO VIBRATIONAL RAINDROP TECHNIQUE

Unison (1:1)

OM/OM – centering, rooting and grounding. Always begin Vibrational Raindrop with this interval. Ground yourself first by applying this interval to your own abdomen about 4 inches below the navel at CV-4. A single note sounded in unison quiets the mind, and old memories become available. Used in mantras.

UT/UT – You may also use this unison next, since UT is the frequency to prepare the body to open and accept the rest of the Sacred Solfeggio frequencies. For release on all levels, but especially on the emotional level.

Microtone *this interval is not used in Sacred Solfeggio VRT*

Interval that is less than an equally spaced semitone, which would be 33 Hz for 12 potential intervals in this system. Microtones are necessary to assist one to move away from grounding and center, to move away from a comfort zone in order to explore new possibilities and stimulate expansion and growth from within.

minor 2nd (16:15)

UT/RE – harsh; carrier of considerable energetic potential, propels the mind, body and spirit into action with power and initiative to remove obstacles. This interval is somewhat dissonant, and supports the formation of new boundaries and structures. The minor and Major 2nd both represent the applications of energy toward the manifestation of material form, in other words creating matter from spirit.

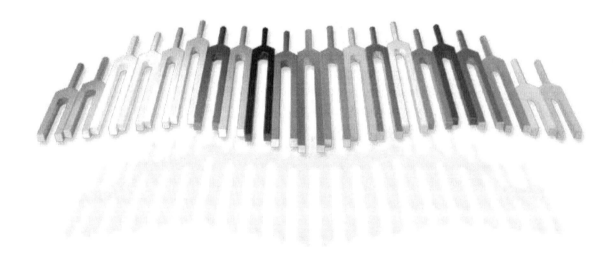

Major 2nd (9:8)

LA/TI – dense but warmer than the minor 2nd; allows access to deep wounds and scars of a physical, emotional, or spiritual nature to transform and repair. Occurs between consonant intervals (octave, 5th, 4th and 3rd) and dissonant intervals (minor 2nd), and thus is the space between harmony and disharmony. Used in modern Classical music.

minor 3rd (6:5)

MI/FA – The minor 3rd reaches more deeply into the emotional level of love and loss. Used in Country Western music. This interval is a baby's first vocal interval: a descending minor 3rd from age 12–15 months. It is the first interval that is learned regardless of culture and may be "encoded" within us. Some examples would be 'Starlight Starbright', the opening of 'Hey Jude' and many more.

Major 3rd (5:4)

RE/MI – optimistic, strength and joy; meditative, dispersive or dispelling effect, relieves mental stress, but is especially useful to relieve physical stress. This interval is used after the Trio of oils in the middle of the VRT session, and it is well-suited to release muscle spasms in the back, especially when used with Aroma Siez®. We use this interval to release stagnant Liver energy, which can be seen in problems such as hot flashes, PMS symptoms, headaches, and anger/frustration issues. Used in Country Western music, Bach.

Perfect 4th (4:3) *The Fourth is the geometric mean of an octave.*

UT/MI; FA/LA – Perfect Fourth; pure, like church bells; stimulates growth, abundance and expansion. Used in Gregorian chant. The Fourth stimulates both sides of the brain; an augmented Fourth is heard in a Tibetan Singing Bowl.

Augmented 4th (45:32)

Earth Star/UT; MI/SOL – highly energetic, full of movement, intense propelling energy, joyful. This interval has been called Crux Ansata, a transition point where spirit is redeemed from matter. This interval is the most fundamental one to build energy and eliminate fatigue. If there is a particular Energy Center (nerve plexus/chakra) that is weak, sound the forks extra times at that level of the spine. An augmented 4th is heard in a Tibetan Singing Bowl.

Perfect 5th (3:2)

FA/TI – The Fifth is the halfway point (harmonic mean) between octaves. A point of release from a particular paradigm; the Fifth moves in all directions. In the key of "C", this would be the notes C and G sounded together. This interval is used in Brazilian music where the interval of the fifth is between the guitar and the voice.

minor 6th (8:5)

UT/FA; MI/LA – mellow sense of longing; tonifies, nourishes beauty, harmony and creative passion but has a quality of inconstancy, desire and yearning for completion. Inversion of the Major Third (4th harmonic of overtone series). A Major Third plus a minor Sixth creates an Octave.

Major 6th (5:3)

Soul Star/Earth Star – optimistic, soft and sweet interval; less emotional than the Major 3rd; builds energy, brings a feeling of fullness and purification; the ultimate expression of Yin. Can bring a sense of magic and fulfillment, with a pull towards healing that allows one's potential to manifest. Known as the Golden Section, Divine Proportion, or Golden Mean. This interval builds yin energy, which moistens, consolidates and cools the body. Heard in lullabies; the sweetest and lightest of intervals.

minor 7th (9:5) *this interval is not used in Sacred Solfeggio VRT*

Major 7th (15:8)

Earth Star/MI; UT/SOL – full of tensions, but not paralyzing like the 2nd; initiative, empowerment, vitalizing and warm, unconditional love; the ultimate expression of Yang. Harsh but more distant, less emotional than the Minor 2nd (its inversion). Strong, warm energy, this interval is used in Raindrop to assist in deletion of old, redundant and useless information so changes can occur and a new order can be achieved. Heard in Beethoven, Ravel and modern jazz (John Coltrane).

Octave (2:1)

Used in all of the "Essential" protocols – Perfect Octave, dreams come true; brings feelings of comfort, completeness, and creates a sense of unity with All That Is.

UT – Emotional Release

RE – Transformation

MI – Miracle DNA

THE PROBLEM OF SACRED SOLFEGGIO INTERVALS

For those of you who already do Vibrational Raindrop Technique with the planetary frequencies, you know that all of the planets have a relationship with the Earth Year (Om) in terms of frequency intervals. In other words, it is a geocentric frequency system. These intervals influence the expression of the planetary forks when used with Om. For instance, Mercury creates a microtone (an interval smaller than a half step) with Om, which gives it the ability to "get between the cracks" especially in terms of communication or when dealing with the shoulders or lungs, which are traditionally Mercury's specific spheres of influence. And as we list each of the planetary frequencies/forks, we see that we have a veritable "Rainbow" of intervals contained within the system. The only missing intervals are the minor 3rd (Nibiru in the Acutonics system fulfills this need), and the Major 7th (fulfilled by Acutonics' Sedna frequency). One could argue whether these planetary intervals are legitimate intervals at all since they are generally not exact, but rather fall within a range of frequency possibilities. In contrast, the Pythagorean frequencies (used by John Beaulieu of Biosonics) and the Tempered Scale with A=440 Hz (used by Fabian Maman of Tama Do) have exact musical and mathematical relationships.

However, the planetary relationship issues mentioned above seem simple when compared with the problem of the Sacred Solfeggio frequencies and intervals. And here's why:

First, the original six Sacred Solfeggio frequencies (396, 417, 528, 639, 741 and 852) cover more than an octave. By definition, the original Sacred Solfeggio octave should range from UT, 396 Hz as the Fundamental to double that, or 792 Hz for the UT', the first octave. Instead, the sixth note, LA, is 852 Hz, already taking us out of the range of our musical octave. This scale might more correctly be called a Pentatonic scale with five notes in the octave. The most common types of pentatonic scales use Major seconds and minor thirds, with no half steps.

As you will see below, it is the Perfect Fourth and Augmented Fourth which are most commonly found in the Sacred Solfeggio scale. You might think it could be called a hexachord scale since there are six notes, but the final note, LA=852 Hz, is outside the theoretic octave frequency of 792 Hz.

But let's put this first problem to the side for now. If we work out the interval relationships of the frequencies, there is no "rainbow" of frequencies to be found. Instead there are some interesting frequency relationships that are seen repeatedly between the notes: a Perfect 4th and an Augmented 4th. For instance, UT (396 Hz) and MI (528 Hz) have a relationship of a Perfect 4th, exactly. Take 396 (UT), multiply x 4 and divide by 3 to get 528, or MI for the 4:3 Just scale Perfect 4th relationship. So that creates a harmony between the First/Root NEC (UT) and the Third/Solar Plexus NEC (MI). (NEC= Neuro- Endocine Center, or Chakra).

There is a second Perfect 4th relationship hidden within the Sacred Solfeggio frequencies: FA (639 Hz) creates a Perfect 4th with LA (852 Hz). That creates a harmony between the Fourth/Heart NEC and the Sixth/Brow NEC. MI (528 Hz) creates almost a "perfect" Augmented 4th with SOL (741 Hz), being 1.5 Hz over (742.5). But for such a large scaled octave (396 Hz), a 1.5 Hz discrepancy is probably okay. In this large scale, each half tone would be worth about 33 Hz, and each Hz might be worth about 3.3 cents, making 1.5 Hz be approximately 4.95 cents. It is said that anything over 5 cents off can be heard as discordant, and this is under 5 cents.

There are other interval relationships possible between all of the nine Sacred Solfeggio frequencies, and all have slight deviancies of 5-10 Hz. However, with intention and other frequencies tools (essential oils, color/light, and so on), one can find many ways to integrate and unify the healing message. They are described in the section on specific intervals in the Sacred Solfeggio system.

MI-SOL and SI-UT: the two whole step intervals

In the "diabolus in musica", the "fa" and "sol" refer to the fourth and fifth notes in a diatonic scale. While all the other notes within the scale transition from one to the other by half steps, it is only between the fourth and fifth notes that the transition is by a whole step.

When talking about intervals, Gurdjieff said, "In *an ascending octave the first 'interval' comes between Mi and Fa. If corresponding additional energy enters at this point the octave will develop without hindrance to Si (Ti), but between Si and Do it needs a much stronger 'additional shock' for its right development than between Mi and Fa, because the vibrations of the octave at this point are of a considerably higher pitch and to overcome a check in the development of the octave a greater intensity is needed."*

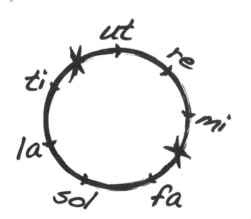

What does this mean? In the drawings that accompany Gurdjieff's notes, he shows the gap that exists between Mi, the third note and Fa, the fourth note. This is the leap that takes us out of our lower emotions up to the "heart-centered view." Once there, we must still take action to move up to the fifth note into the higher emotions, and this is a potentially extremely difficult transition. This is where the energy of the Augmented 4th can be useful to create the dissonance that will propel movement upward. To say it another way, if the notes relate to the Neuro-Endocrine Centers (chakras), then Gurdjieff is talking about the movement upward from the 3rd NEC to the 5th NEC—which, of necessity must involve successful transition through the 4th NEC. Extra energy is needed from outside the system in order to move from the third note (Mi) to the fifth note (SOL) and this extra energy must enter through FA, the 4th NEC.

Because of the uneven frequencies of our Sacred Solfeggio scale, in our system the equivalent Mi/Fa interval would actually be the MI/SOL interval. If each of the frequencies are associated with one of the Neuro-Endocrine Centers, then UT relates to the 1st NEC, RE to the 2nd NEC, and MI to the 3rd NEC, which are the three Neuro-Endocrine centers associated with the denser energy bodies: the physical, the etheric and the lower emotional.

FA is related to the 4th NEC, the Heart Center, the bridge between the Lower Emotional Body, seat of fear and its related emotions, and the Upper Emotional Body, seat of love and its related emotions. Recall that the electric field of the Heart is 60 times greater than the brain and its magnetic field is 5000 times greater than the brain's field (Heart Math)! This is the field (the musical interval) where we decide whether to experience fear-related emotions of the 3rd NEC or love-derived emotions of the 5th NEC.

The MI/SOL interval stretches us from the lower, limiting emotions of material existence up to the emotional freedom of love and joy-derived emotions of the spiritual existence, driven by FA on the way.

The sixth note, LA, relates to the 6th NEC of the Mental Body and inner vision. Interestingly, the fourth note, FA, has a Perfect 4th interval with LA, meaning that the Heart center and the Brow center frequencies can be used together to assist in the harmonious movement upward.

And again, we see this leap of an entire step when we move from the seventh note (SI or TI) to the eighth note, the octave (DO, or UT in the Sacred Solfeggio system). This would be the leap from the realm of the 7th NEC, the Spirit Body, to the many Energy Centers above our material bodies.

When one seeks to expand the consciousness and draw closer to God, one of the paths sometimes chosen is to awaken the potential energy stored within the 1st NEC, coiled at the base of the spine. Some say that it can be found in the sacrum bone and accessed through the Ba

Liao. Activating the Microcosmic Orbit can result in the ability to meditate deeply and experience enlightenment and bliss.

But to awaken this potential energy, one faces the task of unraveling the Three Knots: the First, Fourth and Sixth NECS/Chakras. In terms of the Microcosmic Orbit, these knots would be similar to the three dantians that are encountered in its circuit. These dantians (elixir fields) act as furnaces, where the types of energy in the body (jing, qi and shen) are progressively refined. The base dantian is the most well-known but there is also a dantian located at the heart and another is between the eyebrows. The base dantian transforms essence, or jing, into qi energy. The middle dantian in the middle of the chest transforms qi energy into shen, or spirit, and the higher dantian at the level of the forehead, transforms Shen into wuji, infinite space of void.

If you would like to learn more about how to use these intervals in this method, please consider taking training in Raindrop Harmonics.

CLASSIC AND BODY SYSTEMS
QUICK GUIDE FORKS AND OILS

All of the Systems use the basic Sacred Solfeggio Classic Kit, which includes 10 forks: Low UT, Mid UT (x 2 forks), High UT, Mid MI, Mid SOL, Mid TI, High RE, High FA, and High LA. The core essential oils are different for each System except they all include V6, Ortho Ease® and Aroma Siez®. Metabolic Essentials uses Citrus Cel-Lite Magic® blend in place of Ortho Ease®.

Complete Sacred Angel

Forks:

Complete Sacred Solfeggio x 4 octaves
(All 9 frequencies in 4 octaves)

Essential Oils

*Sacred Angel® (*or White Angelica®)	
Myrrh/Hyssop	Frankincense
Rose/Angelica	Idaho Blue Spruce
Coriander	Melissa/Sandalwood
Geranium	Ylang Ylang

Bible Oils

Forks:

Low UT	Mid UT x 2	Mid MI
Mid SOL	Mid TI	High RE
High FA	High LA	High UT

Essential Oils

Three Wise Men®	Cedarwood/Onycha
Hyssop	Galbanum/Sandalwood
Myrtle	Cistus/Cassia
Spikenard/Myrrh	Frankincense
Cypress	

Brain

Forks:

Low UT	Mid UT x 2	Mid MI
Mid SOL	Mid TI	High RE
High FA	High LA	High UT

Essential Oils

Valor®	Cardamom
Oregano	M-Grain®
Thyme	Peace & Calming®
Clarity®	Peppermint

Classic

Forks:

Low UT	Mid UT x 2	Mid MI
Mid SOL	Mid TI	High RE
High FA	High LA	High UT

Essential Oils

Valor®	Wintergreen
Oregano	Marjoram
Thyme	Cypress
Basil	Peppermint

Colon & Digestion

Forks:

Low UT	Mid UT x 2	Mid MI
Mid SOL	Mid TI	High RE
High FA	High LA	High UT

Essential Oils

Valor®	Tarragon
Oregano	Di-Gizer®
Thyme	Fennel
Cumin	Spearmint

Heart/Circulation

Forks:

Low UT	Mid UT x 2	Mid MI
Mid SOL	Mid TI	High RE
High FA	High LA	High UT

Essential Oils

Valor®	Clove
Oregano	Aroma Lifer®
Thyme	Cypress
Goldenrod	Nutmeg

Hormone Balance/Female

Forks:

Low UT	Mid UT x 2	Mid MI
Mid SOL	Mid TI	High RE
High FA	High LA	High UT

Essential Oils

Valor®	Fleabane
Oregano	EndoFlex®
Thyme	Clary Sage
Dragon Time®	Peppermint

Hormone Balance/Male

Forks:

Low UT	Mid UT x 2	Mid MI
Mid SOL	Mid TI	High RE
High FA	High LA	High UT

Essential Oils

Valor®	Bluc Yarrow
Oregano	Mister®
Thyme	Myrtle
Lavender	Peppermint

Joints & Bones

Forks:

Low UT	Mid UT x 2	Mid MI
Mid SOL	Mid TI	High RE
High FA	High LA	High UT

Essential Oils

Valor®	Wintergreen
Oregano	Panaway®
Thyme	Spruce
Helichrysum	Peppermint

Liver

Forks:

Low UT	Mid UT x 2	Mid MI
Mid SOL	Mid TI	High RE
High FA	High LA	High UT

Essential Oils

Valor®	German Chamomile
Oregano	Juvaflex®
Thyme	Ledum
Carrot Seed	Peppermint

Longevity

Forks:

Low UT	Mid UT x 2	Mid MI
Mid SOL	Mid TI	High RE
High FA	High LA	High UT

Essential Oils

Valor®	Clove
Oregano	Longevity®
Thyme	Frankincense
Orange	Peppermint

Lung

Forks:

Low UT	Mid UT x 2	Mid MI
Mid SOL	Mid TI	High RE
High FA	High LA	High UT

Essential Oils

Valor®	Melrose®
Oregano Raven®	
Thyme Myrtle	
Eucalyptus Radiata Ravensara	

Sacred Angel

Forks:

Low UT	Mid UT x 2	Mid MI
Mid SOL	Mid TI	High RE
High FA	High LA	High UT

Essential Oils

*Sacred Angel® (*or White Angelica®)	
Myrrh/Hyssop	Frankincense
Rose/Angelica	Idaho Blue Spruce
Coriander	Melissa/Sandalwood
Geranium	Ylang Ylang

SACRED ANGEL
Sacred Solfeggio Vibrational Raindrop Technique
QUICK REFERENCE RAINDROP OUTLINE

Forks:		Essential Oils	
Low UT	High UT	*Sacred Angel® (*or White Angelica®)	
Mid UT x 2	High RE	Myrrh/Hyssop	Frankincense
Mid MI	High FA	Rose/Angelica	Idaho Blue Spruce
Mid SOL	High LA	Coriander	Melissa/Sandalwood
Mid TI	OM Unison	Geranium	Ylang Ylang

1. **Facilitator: Apply White Angelica to self on shoulders, back of neck, thymus.**
   Apply Om Unison to self at CV-4 (Origin Pass) for grounding.

2. **HAVE CLIENT LIE FACE UP. ESTABLISH ENERGY BALANCE:**
   Listen to UT Unison (2 UT forks) (hold tuning forks at least 6" from client's ears).
   Sacred Angel®: Rub on Shoulders (1-2 drops/shoulder) and Feet (1-2 drops/foot),
   R hand/R foot, L hand/L foot; R hand/R shoulder, L hand/L shoulder.
   Hold until you feel the energy balance left and right.
   Apply UT Unison (1 UT fork to the sole of each foot) at KI-1 (Gushing Spring).

3. **VIBRATIONAL VITA FLEX on Spinal Reflex Area of Feet** (1-3 drops each oil to each foot)

HYSSOP	FRANKINCENSE	ANGELICA
I.B. SPRUCE	CORIANDER	SANDALWOOD
GERANIUM	YLANG YLANG	

   Apply the Low UT Octave (UT and Low UT forks) with Low UT at CV-4 (Origin Pass) on the abdomen four finger-widths below the umbilicus, and UT at CV-17 (Chest Center) in the center of the chest level with the 4th rib. Then apply the Low UT Octave (UT and Low UT forks) with Low UT at CV-17 (Chest Center) and UT at GV-24.5 (Yin Tang) between the eyebrows.
   - HAVE CLIENT ROLL OVER TO A FACE DOWN POSITION

4. **HYSSOP (MYRRH):** Raindrop V-6 (6" above) 4-6 drops from sacrum to atlas.
   Myrrh (1 drop) at GV-4 and activate in clockwise direction.
   Raindrop (6" above) 1-2 drops Hyssop from sacrum to atlas.
   Feather stroke 3" straight up spine. Repeat with 6" then 12" strokes.
   FRANKINCENSE: Raindrop (6" above) 1-2 drops from sacrum to atlas.
   Feather stroke 3" straight up spine. Repeat with 6" then 12" strokes.
   Feather straight to sides in each position.
   Feather with full length strokes up and out, off the shoulders.
   Apply the Mid UT/Mid TI interval (Mid UT and Mid TI forks) with the Mid UT fork on GV2 (Low Back Shu)

at base of sacrum and the Mid TI fork on GV-11 (Spirit Path) below T-5. Next apply the Mid TI 7th (Mid UT and Mid TI forks) with the Mid UT fork on GV-11 (Spirit Path) and the Mid TI fork on GV20 (Hundred Convergences) at the crown of the head.

5. ANGELICA (ROSE), CORIANDER, and IDAHO BLUE SPRUCE

Apply Rose at GV-11 (similar to Myrrh as in Step 4.)

Raindrop and feather each other oil on spine, as in Step 4 (HYSSOP). .

Finger circles (after all three oils are applied).

Apply the Mid UT/Mid MI interval (Mid UT and Mid MI forks) to the band of muscles next to the spine, right side first. Walk up this band with the forks, moving about 2-3" each time. When completed, apply one fork at the bottom of the band and one fork at the top of the band.

Apply Mid MI 3rd (Mid UT and Mid MI forks) wherever muscle knots are found.

6. SANDALWOOD (MELISSA)

Apply Melissa at GV-16 (similar to Myrrh as in Step 4.)

Raindrop and feather Sandalwood on spine, as in Step 4 (HYSSOP). .

Feather stroke 3" straight up spine. Repeat with 6" then 12" strokes.

Thumb Vitaflex up spine.

Saw Maneuver up spine.

Stretch and Quiver up spine.

Apply the Mid UT/Mid SOL Interval (Mid UT and Mid SOL forks) on the Huato Jiaji points up the spine from sacrum to base of skull, alternating the Mid UT and Mid SOL forks on either side of the spine. The Huato Jiaji points are found on either side of the spine between the vertebrae.

7. ORTHO EASE®

Apply to entire back, followed by large circles with palms.

Palm Slide up & down the back. Apply more Ortho Ease® if needed.

Sound the High UT/High FA Interval (High UT and High FA forks) above the spine in DN-8 move from sacrum to crown, then one straight sweep down and off the feet.

8. GERANIUM

Sprinkle (6" above) from sacrum to atlas.

Feather stroke 3" straight up spine. Repeat with 6" then 12" strokes.

Arched feather stroke 3" straight up spine. Repeat with 6" then 12" strokes.

Feather with full length strokes up and out, off the shoulders.

Sound the High UT/High RE Interval (High UT and High RE forks) above the spine in DN-8 move from sacrum to crown, then one straight sweep down and off the feet.

9. YLANG YLANG

Raindrop (6" above) 1-2 drops from sacrum to atlas. Feather as with Geranium.

10. WARM COMPRESS

Apply alternating layers of dry-wet-dry towels to client's back and pull sheet up over towels

Sound the High UT/High LA interval in the shape of a Tetrahedron (GV-20, PC-8 and GV-11 as anchor points). Tap the forks together over the body GV-11 (Spirit Path), then move the High LA fork to GV-20 (Hundred Convergences) while the High UT fork stays above GV-11. Bring the forks together again above GV-11, then separate and take the forks to PC-8 (Construction Palace), one fork above each of the palms. Bring the forks together again above GV-11, tap them, and take them together down to GV-20, separate them so that each fork goes to one of the palms above PC-8, and bring them together between the palms (over the sacrum), then back up to starting position above GV-11.

Apply the Low UT Octave (Low UT and Mid UT forks) to the sole of each foot at KI-1 (Gushing Spring).

11 & 12   EVALUATE AND GIVE WATER

ESSENTIALS
Sacred Solfeggio Vibrational Raindrop Technique

Forks:

Low UT   OM Unison
Mid UT x 2
High UT
(or whatever Essential Kit is being used)

Essential Oils

Valor®   White Angelica
Oils for the System being used

1. **Facilitator: Apply White Angelica to self on shoulders, back of neck, thymus.**
   Apply Om Unison to self at CV-4 (Origin Pass) for grounding.

2. **HAVE CLIENT LIE FACE UP. ESTABLISH ENERGY BALANCE:**
   Listen to UT Unison (2 UT forks) (hold tuning forks at least 6" from client's ears).
   VALOR®: Rub on Shoulders (1-2 drops/shoulder) and Feet (1-2 drops/foot),
   R hand/R foot, L hand/L foot; R hand/R shoulder, L hand/L shoulder.
   Hold until you feel the energy balance left and right.
   Apply UT Unison (1 UT fork to the sole of each foot) at KI-1 (Gushing Spring).

3. **VIBRATIONAL VITA FLEX on Spinal Reflex Area of Feet** (1-3 drops each oil to each foot)
   OIL #1   OIL #2   OIL #3
   OIL #4   OIL #5   OIL #7
   Apply the Low UT Octave (UT and Low UT forks) with Low UT at CV-4 (Origin Pass) on the abdomen four finger-widths below the umbilicus, and UT at CV-17 (Chest Center) in the center of the chest level with the 4th rib. Then apply the Low UT Octave (UT and Low UT forks) with Low UT at CV-17 (Chest Center) and UT at GV-24.5 (Yin Tang) between the eyebrows.
   • HAVE CLIENT ROLL OVER TO A FACE DOWN POSITION

4. **OIL #1: Raindrop V-6** (6" above) 4-6 drops from sacrum to atlas.
   Raindrop (6" above) 1-2 drops Oil #1 from sacrum to atlas.
   Feather stroke 3" straight up spine. Repeat with 6" then 12" strokes.
   OIL #2: Raindrop (6" above) 1-2 drops Oil #2 from sacrum to atlas.
   Feather stroke 3" straight up spine. Repeat with 6" then 12" strokes.
   Feather straight to sides in each position.
   Feather with full length strokes up and out, off the shoulders.
   Apply the Mid UT/Mid TI interval (Mid UT and Mid TI forks) with the Mid UT fork on GV2 (Low Back Shu) at base of sacrum and the Mid TI fork on GV-11 (Spirit Path) below T-5. Next apply the Mid TI 7th (Mid UT and Mid TI forks) with the Mid UT fork on GV-11 (Spirit Path) and the Mid TI fork on GV20 (Hundred Convergences) at the crown of the head.

5. OIL #3, OIL #4, and OIL #5

Raindrop and feather each oil on spine, as in Step 4 (Oil #1).

Finger circles (after all three oils are applied).

Apply the Mid UT Unison (two Mid UT forks) to the band of muscles next to the spine, right side first. Walk up this band with the forks, moving about 2-3" each time. When completed, apply one fork at the bottom of the band and one fork at the top of the band.

Apply Mid UT Unison (two Mid UT forks) wherever muscle knots are found.

6. OIL #6

Sprinkle (6" above) from sacrum to atlas.

Feather stroke 3" straight up spine. Repeat with 6" then 12" strokes.

Thumb Vitaflex up spine.

Saw Maneuver up spine.

Stretch and Quiver up spine.

Apply the Mid UT Unison (two Mid UT forks) on the Huato Jiaji points up the spine from sacrum to base of skull. The Huato Jiaji points are found on either side of the spine between the vertebrae.

7. ORTHO EASE®

Apply to entire back, followed by large circles with palms.

Palm Slide up & down the back. Apply more Ortho Ease® if needed.

Apply the UT Octaves (Low UT with Mid UT forks; then Mid UT with High UT forks, then High UT with Angelic UT forks) to the Neuro-Endocrine centers/Chakras. First Apply the Low UT and Mid UT forks to the Root/1st Chakra at GV-2 at the same time. Next apply the Mid UT fork at GV-2 and sound the High UT fork around the weighted end of the Mid UT fork in a clockwise direction spiraling upward, and finally sound the High UT and Angelic UT above GV-2. Repeat this for each of the Neuro-Endocrine centers on the spine, moving to GV-4, GV-6, GV-11, GV-14, GV-16 and GV-20.

8. VALOR®

Sprinkle (6" above) from sacrum to atlas.

Feather stroke 3" straight up spine. Repeat with 6" then 12" strokes.

Arched feather stroke 3" straight up spine. Repeat with 6" then 12" strokes.

Feather with full length strokes up and out, off the shoulders.

Sound the High UT Octave (High UT and Angelic UT forks) above the spine in DN-8 move from sacrum to crown, then one straight sweep down and off the feet.

9. OIL #7

Raindrop (6" above) 1-2 drops from sacrum to atlas. Feather as with Valor.

10. WARM COMPRESS

Apply alternating layers of dry-wet-dry towels to client's back and pull sheet up over towels

Sound the High UT Octave (High UT and Angelic UT forks) in the shape of a Tetrahedron (GV-20, PC-8 and GV-11 as anchor points). Tap the forks together over the body GV-11 (Spirit Path), then move the Angelic UT fork to GV-20 (Hundred Convergences) while the High UT fork stays above GV-11. Bring the forks together again above GV-11, then separate and take the forks to PC-8 (Construction Palace), one fork above each of the palms. Bring the forks together again above GV-11, tap them, and take them together down to GV-20, separate them so that each fork goes to one of the palms above PC-8, and bring them together between the palms (over the sacrum), then back up to starting position above GV-11.

Apply the Low UT Octave (Low UT and Mid UT forks) to the sole of each foot at KI-1 (Gushing Spring).

11 & 12   EVALUATE AND GIVE WATER

MESOCOSM: Pythagorean Frequencies and Vibrational Raindrop Technique (PYVRT)

Pythagorean Tuning

Pythagorean tuning is a system of tuning that focuses on specific frequency intervals. Based on Pythagoras's view of music as a microcosm of the world in which we live, it uses a system of pitch and rhythm that is ruled by the same mathematical laws that govern the universe/macrocosm. "As above, so below."

Disease manifests in the physical, Newtonian world in which we live. But its root causes are in the nonphysical, Quantum world. The Pythagorean frequencies (body) are the link between the Sacred Solfeggio (mind) and the Planetary (spirit).

The ancient Greeks felt that music had a moral quality and therefore an important effect on people and nature. Pythagorus (c. 582-507 BCE) was born in Ionia on the island of Sámos, and eventually settled in Crotone, a Dorian Greek colony in southern Italy, in 529 B.C.E. Very little is known about him, except he lectured in philosophy and mathematics. He also started an academy which gradually formed into a society or brotherhood called the *Order of the Pythagoreans.*

He is said to have had his first musical "aha" experience when he was walking past a blacksmith shop, where they were hammering metal. Pythagoras observed that when the blacksmith struck his anvil, different notes were produced according to the weight of the hammer. Being interested in string instruments, he performed various experiments and came up with a scale that sounds more or less normal to our ears, but the scale is not exactly the same everywhere. Number (in this case *amount of weight*) seemed to govern musical tone.

According to Greek historical tradition, Pythagoras went on to build a monochord. He asked himself what a 1:1 ratio sounds like and plucked the monochord; then plucked it a second time. Next Pythagoras divided the string in half and compared the sound produced by half the string to the sound of the original full string. In so doing, he heard what a 2:1 ratio sounds like: an octave. The octave is an acoustical phenomenon that has been used in music for hundreds, if not thousands, of years. Pythagoras correctly identified the octave as the sonic manifestation of the simplest of all numerical ratios: 2:1, known as a *Diapason* (Greek) meaning "through all the tones."

At some point in his life, Pythagoras had an epiphany: the simpler the numerical ratio between vibrating bodies, the more blended and, therefore, the more consonant the interval (an interval can be defined as the sonic relationship between vibrating bodies). This realization led towards his own developing belief that the universe and everything in it could be explained through **numbers**. The central doctrine of the Pythagoreans, in fact, was "a belief in the importance of numbers as a guide to the interpretation of the world." *(The New Grove Dictionary of Music and Musicians, Vol.15, page 485)*

Next he divided the monochord into thirds, and compared the sound made by half the string with the sound made by a third of the string (2:3). It was powerful and beautiful, and we now know it as the Perfect Fifth (*Diapente* in Greek).

Even though the two pitches do not blend together into a single pitch, there is minimal "third force" (extra sounds) in this interval. It is called a Fifth because the second pitch (1/3 of the string) is five diatonic steps above the pitch created by the sound of half of the string.

Finally, Pythagoras divided the monochord into quarters and compared the sound made by a quarter of the string with a third of the string (4:3), called the Perfect Fourth (*Diatessaron* in Greek). While it was slightly more complex than the Fifth, it was still harmonious. Pythagorus developed what may be the first completely mathematically based scale which resulted by considering intervals of the octave (a factor of 2 in frequency) and intervals of fifths (a factor of 3/2 in frequency). The scale was perfect, and contained four fifths and five fourths in its diatonic (8 note) scale.

Thus, the essential, or Prime intervals, were discovered and described. They are Perfect: Unison (Tonic), Octave, Fifth (Dominant) and Fourth (Subdominant). Most significantly, the Pythagoreans found that these pleasant intervals could be expressed as the ratio of whole numbers.

Ratio	Name	Interval	Greek term	Latin term
6:12	octave	(1:2)	diapson	duplus
6:9 or 8:12	fourth	(2:3)	diapente	desquiltera
6:8 or 9:12	fifth	(3:4)	diatessaron	sequitertia
1:1	tone	(1:1)	tonus	- - -

Plato described many of the concepts of the Pythagoreans, which is why we know as much as we do today. Music is:

Heard by the Ear,
Registered in the Brain,
Carried to the Blood,
Transmitted to the Soul.

Music was considered to be such a powerful influence on health that healing centers of Asclepeion at Pergamum and Epidauros in Greece used music to accompany their therapies. And Boethius (480-524 CE) said that the soul and the body are subject to the same laws of proportion that govern music and the cosmos itself.

Aristotle (Plato's student) said, *"The (Pythagoreans were) ... the first to take up mathematics ... (and) thought its principles were the principles of all things. Since, of these principles, numbers ... are the first, ... in numbers they seemed to see many resemblances to things that exist ... more than [just] air, fire and earth and water, (but things such as) justice, soul, reason, opportunity ..." "[the Pythagoreans] saw that the ... ratios of musical scales were expressible in numbers [and that] .. all things seemed to be modeled on numbers, and numbers seemed to be the first things in the whole of nature, they supposed the elements of number to be the elements of all things, and the whole heaven to be a musical scale and a number."*

The Pythagoreans were certain that the distances between the planets would have the same harmonious ratios that they could hear in a plucked string. They thought the solar system consisted of ten spheres revolving around a central fire, and each sphere/planet made a sound as it moved through the air. The closer spheres gave lower tones while the more distant moved faster and gave higher pitched sounds; all of it combining into a heavenly harmony, the "music of the spheres."

Plato developed this idea, and described the cosmos in his Republic: *". . . Upon each of its circles stood a siren who was carried round with its movements, uttering the concords of a single scale..."* In the Timaeus, he describes the circles of heaven subdivided according to the musical ratios.

20 centuries later, Kepler wrote in his *Harmonice Munde* (1619) that he wished *"...to erect the magnificent edifice of the harmonic system of the musical scale . . . as God, the Creator Himself, has expressed it in harmonizing the heavenly motions."* And later, *"I grant you that no sounds are given forth, but I affirm . . . that the movements of the planets are modulated according to harmonic proportions."* Planetary VRT frequencies were calculated by Kepler, then brought to audible frequencies by Cousto in the 1970s (via the Law of the Octave). But the concept of "planetary sounds" originated with the Pythagoreans.

Pythagorean Scales

What is a Pythagorean scale? This can be a tricky question to answer unless you approach it from the point of view of numbers. Remember that Pythagoras thought that the world of numbers was the source of creation, and that he believed that Prime numbers were the essence of life. But he limited his scale definition to include only numbers that were divisible by 2 and/or 3.

Pythagorean scale   [pə,thag·ə′rē·ən ′skāl]
A musical scale such that the frequency intervals are represented by the ratios of integral powers of the numbers 2 and 3   http://encyclopedia2.thefreedictionary.com/Pythagorean+scale

The Pythagorean scale is generated from just two integers (2 and 3). Multiplying the frequency of any tone by 2 produces the characteristic sound of an octave, and multiplying by 3 then dividing by 2 produces the characteristic sound of a "fifth" (the fifth tone in the diatonic scale: Do Re Mi Fa Sol).

In other words, a Pythagorean scale can start with any frequency, such as 128 Hz. As an example, ne then calculates the rest of the scale with the following results.

Note	Our Pythagorean scale example	Pythagorean Ratio to Fundamental
C	1.000 = 128	1.000
D	9/8 = 144	9/8 = 1.1.25
E	81/64 = 161.92	81/64 = 1.2656
F	4/3 = 170.66	4/3 = 1.3333
G	3/2 = 192	3/2 = 1.5
A	27/16 = 216	27/16 = 1.6875
B	243/128 = 242.99	243/128 = 1.8984
C	2.000 = 256	2.000

Using 2 and 3 as our fundamental numbers, look at each fraction of the scale and you can break it down to 2 and 3.
3/2 is 3/2 (Fifth),
3/4 is 3/2x2 (Fourth),
9/8 is 3x3/2x2x2 (Second),
27/16 is 3x3x3/2x2x2x2 (Sixth),
81/64 is 3x3x3x3/2x2x2x2x2x2 (Third), and
243/128 is 3x3x3x3x3/2x2x2x2x2x2x2 (Seventh).

By contrast, in a Just Scale, other whole numbers are allowed, such as 5, and is more commonly used in modern non-tempered scales.

All of the 8 pitches of the Pythagorean diatonic scale are produced by repeatedly multiplying by 3/2 until you reach a tone close to an octave of the original. The word "diatonic" is Greek and means "proceeding by whole tones." Pythagorean tuning is a spiral, on open loop of Perfect Fifths (3:2), and looks like a nautilus spiral.

Pythagorean VRT Scale

For the trinity of VRT Tuning Systems, the Pythagorean Scale has 126 Hz as its fundamental (rather than 128 Hz). The interval calculations generally follow typical Pythagorean ratios as described above, except for Factor 9 tuning used in the cases of sharps and flats. This is how it looks with the frequencies of the forks which are in the Pythagorean Classic VRT Kit highlighted and the Fundamental in bold:

Note	Low	Mid	High	Angelic
C	63	**126**	252	504
C#	67.5	135	270	540
D	72	144	288	576
D#	76.5	153	306	612
E	81	162	324	643
F	85.5	171	342	684
F#	90	180	360	720
G	94.5	189	378	756
G#	99	198	396	792
Ab	103.5	207	414	828
A	108	216	432	864
A#	112.5	225	450	900
B	117	234	456	936

Currently, we use only the Pythagorean Classic tuning forks, but will be teaching classes about how to integrate this system with the Sacred Solfeggio via UT (396 Hz), how to integrate this system with the Planetary frequency via the Sun (126 Hz), and the rich collection of sacred geometry frequencies embedded within this table!

Special Considerations

HOW TO HANDLE TUNING FOrKS

For the best vibration, hold the tuning fork at its throat, where the prongs meet the stem, and firmly tap it on your Leg Activator or Table Top Activator. The less you touch the prongs, the longer the vibration you will have. With a bent elbow, relaxed arm and flick of the wrist, strike only one weight on the tuning fork (or one prong on the unweighted tuning fork) at a 3/4 angle for the best vibration. If you observe closely, you will see both tips of the fork prongs vibrating slightly as they visibly demonstrate a sound wave.

You may now apply the stem of the weighted tuning fork to the point on the body where desired. If the fork is unweighted, you may now move it above the physical body in the various energy body fields, as desired. In both cases, you are transferring the sound wave and its energy to the physical body and/or biofield.

Some Concerns or Contraindications to the use of Tuning Forks with Essential Oils
- Drug or alcohol intoxication
- Certain medications may reduce effectiveness, such as corticosteroids, benzodiazepines, or narcotics
- Use of a pacemaker
- Hearing aids (these should be removed)
- A seizure disorder
- Bleeding disorder such as hemophilia, or the use of blood thinners
- Infections and open wounds, skin disorders or disease
- Pregnancy
- Allergy to metal (tuning forks are usually aluminum)

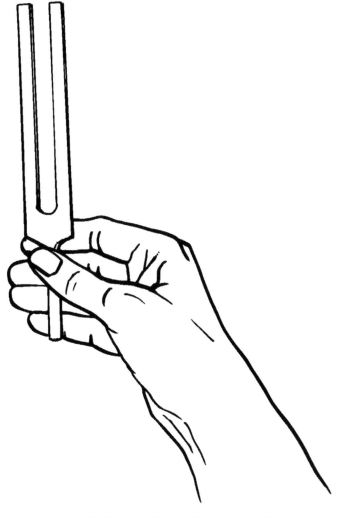

HOLDING TUNING FORK

OCTAVES OF FORKS

Low-frequency forks are used to reach a deeper level of healing with the forks. They reach into the cellular DNA level of healing.

Mid-frequency forks are weighted in order to provide vibration that is dense enough to affect the physical body on which they are applied. At times they may be held near the ears for the benefit of the client, but usually no closer than 6 inches. Remove hearing aids before sounding forks near the ears.

High frequency forks are non-weighted, and are meant to primarily affect the subtle bodies (etheric, emotional, mental, spiritual and other fields). They should usually not be sounded closer than 12" from the body because the energy fields are above and around the physical body. I personally will sound them about 24" above and around the client. In general, avoid sounding them around the client's head to avoid client discomfort.

THREE OCTAVES OF FORKS

You may use 3 octaves of an interval rather than just the single interval that is described in the protocol. For instance, instead of using only the Om and Neptune forks to create a 5th Interval while working on the Huato Jiaji along the spine, you may do the following:

First apply the Low Om and the Low Neptune forks to the Huato Jiaji points. Next apply the Om and Neptune forks to these points. Finally sound the High Om and High Neptune above the Huato Jiaji points as you move the forks up the spine. In this way, you have connected your intention from the physical body to the subtle bodies.

Special Techniques

The **"DN-8"** movement is a special way of sounding high frequency forks that emerged while blending the use of tuning forks with Raindrop Technique. It involves making small Figure 8's above the client, but alternating which of your wrists is above the other when they come together for the middle and beginning/end of the Figure 8. It resonates with the morphic field of the helical structure of DNA.

Relaxing Muscle Spasms: Here is an excellent way to relax the entire band of muscles that runs along the spine on either side:

Apply the Om forks to the band of muscles about 1.5" out from the spine on each side just above the hip. "Walk up" this band with the forks, moving about 2"-3" each time. Have Fork #1 move up 2"-3" then Fork #2 joins it; and the process is repeated up the entire band of muscles. When done, apply one fork to each end of the band (one near the shoulder and one near the hip). Repeat on other side. This technique can be used on other tight muscles, such as the IT band on the thigh.

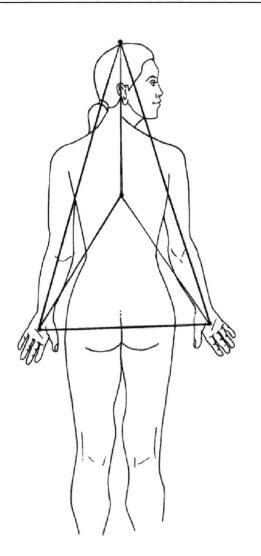

The **"Benediction"** sequence used in Step 10 of both the Bible Oils and the Metabolic Essentials VRT is based on the points used in Acutonics' Cosmic Capstone (GV20, CV17 and PC8), which in turn is based on Esoteric Acupuncture's Integration Synthesis Pattern. The Facilitator creates the sacred geometry of a Tetrahedron with the tuning forks over the Receiver:

Sound the High Om Octave (High Om-1 and Angelic Om) in the shape of a Tetrahedron (GV20, PC8 and GV11 as anchor points). Tap the forks together over the body about 24"above GV11 (Spirit Path), then move one fork to GV20 (Hundred Convergences) while the other fork stays above GV11. Bring the forks together again above GV11, then separate and take each fork to PC8 (Construction Palace), one fork above each of the palms. Bring the forks together again about 24" above GV11, take them together down to GV20, separate them so that each fork goes to one of the palms above PC8, and bring them together between the palms, then back up to starting position above GV11. Repeat x 3.

Amount of oils: use V-6 to dilute and/or decrease number of drops of essential oil.

Selected Bibliography

Beaulieu, John, *Human Tuning*, New York, NY: Biosonic Enterprises, 2010

Beaulieu, John, *Music and Sound in the Healing Arts*, Barrytown, NY: Station Hill Press, 1987

Berendt, Joachim-Ernst, *The World is Sound, Nada Brahma,* Rochester, VT: Destiny Books, 1883

Burroughs, Stanley, *Healing for the Age of Enlightenment,* Newcastle, CA: 1976

Carey, Donna, and de Muynk, Marjorie, Acutonics: *There's no place like Om,* Vadito, NM: Devachan Press, 2002

Carey, Donna, et.al., *Acutonics: From Galaxies to Cells,* Llano, NM: Devachan Press, 2010

Chia, Mantak, *Healing Light of the Tao,* Rochester, VT: Destiny Books, 1993

Cousto, Hans, *The Cosmic Octave: Origin of Harmony,* Mendocino, CA: LifeRhythm, 2000

de Muynck, Marjorie, *Sound Healing: Vibrational Healing with Om Tuning Forks,* Santa Fe, NM, Lemniscate Music, 2008

Elliott, S; Minsum, K; Beaulieu, J; Stefano, G, "Sound therapy induced relaxation: down regulating stress processes and pathologies", Med Sci Monit, 2003; 9(5): RA116-121, as reprinted in *Human Tuning*

Emoto, Masaru, The Hidden Messages in Water, Hillsboro, OR: Beyond Words Publishing, 2004 Goldman, Jonathan, *Shifting Frequencies,* Flagstaff, AZ: Light Technology Publishing, 1998

Goldman, Jonathan, *Healing Sounds: The Power of Harmonics*, Rochester, VT: Healing Arts Press, 1992 Hesse, Hermann, Magister Ludi, New York, NY: Bantam, 1982

Higley, Alan and Connie, *Reference Guide to Essential Oils, Twelfth Edition,* Spanish Fork, UT: Abundant Health, 2010

Jenny, Hans, *Cymatics*, Newmarket, NH: MACROmedia, 2001

Lauterwasser, Alexander, *Water Sound Images*, Newmarket, NH: MACROmedia, 2002

Manwaring, Brian, Ed., *Essential Oils Desk Reference, 4th Edition,* Lehi, UT: Essential Science Publishing, 2009

Prigogine, Ilya, *Order Out of Chaos,* New York, NY: Bantam Books, 1984

Sankey, Mikio, *Esoteric Acupuncture,* Inglewood, CA: Mountain Castle Publishing, 1999

Stewart, David, *A Statistical Validation of Raindrop VIBRATIONAL RAINDROP TECHNIQUE,* Marble Hill, MO: Care Publications, 2003

Stewart, David, *The Chemistry of Essential Oils Made Simple (God's Love Manifest in Molecules),* Marble Hill, MO: Care Publications, 2005 and 2006

Stewart, David, *Quantum Physics, Essential Oils, and the Mind-Body Connection, (How Essential Oils Really Work),* American Fork, UT: Sound Concepts, 2009

Thompson, Oscar, editor, *International Cyclopedia of Music and Musicians, Ninth edition,* New York, NY: Dodd Mead & Company, 1964

Young, D. Gary, *Essential Oils Integrative Medical Guide,* Lehi, UT: Essential Science Publishing, 2006

Young, D. Gary, *Raindrop Technique,,* Lehi, UT: Essential Science Publishing, 2008

Selected Resources

Tuning Forks

For more information about the tuning forks used in this book, please visit www.AromaSounds.com. We have Planetary, Sacred Solfeggio, Pythagorean and other tuning forks made by AromaSounds.

Essential Oils

For more information about Young Living Essential Oils, please visit www.ylwebsite.com/integrativemedky

Classes

Introductory classes on Vibrational Raindrop Technique and Raindrop Harmonics are taught by Certified Raindrop Harmonics Coaches http://www.raindropharmonics.com/Coaches.html and Certified VRT Coaches http://www.vibrationalraindroptechnique.com/meet-our-instructors.html. Check online for up-to-date listings of their classes.

Advanced classes on **Vibrational Raindrop Technique** and **Raindrop Harmonics** are taught by Dr. Christi Bonds-Garrett. Check online for her schedule at http://www.drbondsgarrett.com/calendar.html. These classes are certified by the Natural Therapies Certification Board, www.NTCB.org, and lead to Certification as a Raindrop Harmonics Specialist. Classes are also certified for Continuing Education by the National Certification Board for Therapeutic Massage & Bodywork, www.NCBTMB.org.

Books

VRT Workbook, Available from AromaSounds, 233 North 7th Street, Paducah, KY 42001
- (270) 415-1752 • or visit www.AromaSounds.com

Raindrop Harmonics, Available from AromaSounds, 233 North 7th Street, Paducah, KY 42001
- (270) 415-1752 • or visit www.AromaSounds.com

DVDs

Vibrational Raindrop Technique DVD, Available from AromaSounds, 233 North 7th Street, Paducah, KY 42001 • (270) 415-1752 • or visit www.AromaSounds.com

Raindrop Harmonics DVD, Available from AromaSounds, 233 North 7th Street, Paducah, KY 42001
- (270) 415-1752 • or visit www.AromaSounds.com

CDs

Jonathan Goldman at www.HealingSounds.com
Andrew Weil and Kimba Arem at www.SoundsTrue.com
Marjorie de Muynk at www.SoundsTrue.com

Raindrop Harmonics Certification Program*

Phase 1 –Vibrational Raindrop Technique – Introduction to Body Systems and Vibrational VitaFlex

Review of Vibrational Raindrop Technique (VRT), other vibrational techniques such as Vibrational VitaFlex (VVF) and the use of Essential Oils. Hands on experience with VRT and VVF utilizing the Planetary Classic Tuning Fork Kit and other Systems Kits with Young Living essential oils.

Phase 2 – Vibrational Neuro-Endocrine Centers, Vibrational Neuro-Auricular Technique

Introduction to Neuro-Endocrine Centers, how to access them, and their relationship to the Autonomic Nervous System and the Micro-Cosmic Orbit. Learn to identify and remove blockages from the energy fields of the body using the Essential Om Tuning Fork Kit and Gem Tip tuning forks. Explore Vibrational Auricular Technique and the Crystal Palace of the brain.

Phase 3 – Chromatic Raindrop Technique

Introduction to Light and Color Harmonics, and how to work with color harmonics in Vibrational Raindrop Technique.

Explore how vibrational therapies of sound and light, Neuro-Endocrine Centers and energy healing processes can be integrated into your life and professional practice to enhance therapeutic outcomes.

Learn the anatomy of energy circuits and how they affect your body structure, facilitate emotional release and strengthen mental processes.

Discover the dynamics of sound healing and energy fields, and their application to the body via energy meridian pathways.

Educate yourself, heal yourself and others, and transform your delivery of Wellness care.

All classes are Interactive lecture with multi-media presentations taught by Dr. Christi Bonds-Garrett, developer of Vibrational Raindrop Technique.

*A program of AromaSounds, certified through the Natural Therapies Certification Board www.ntcb.org

Comments

«Dr. Christi Bonds-Garrett wonderfully integrates Acutonics with Vibrational Raindrop Technique, creating a unique synergy between these two powerful modalities. The age of sound and light has truly arrived and is enriched by this new contribution to holistic health care."

Donna Carey, LAc & Ellen F. Franklin, MA
Kairos Institute of Sound Healing, Creators of the Acutonics Healing System

«Dr. Bonds-Garrett is dedicated to the exploration and the application of Vibrational Medicine as a viable form of healing. It is very rare to find a practitioner and scholar who can merge Western Medicine and Vibrational Medicine in a way that is comprehensible and applicable. But she has done this by merging the Acutonics Sound Healing System and Young Living Essential Oils, creating the Vibrational Raindrop Technique.

It has been very inspiring to watch Christi blend these systems, keeping the integrity of each one while masterfully weaving them together. She has created a powerful vibrational healing technique that balances and harmonizes all of the senses.

Dr. Bonds-Garrett is an Energy Medicine Pioneer and it is a true honor working with her."

Susan B. Goldstone, L.Ac, Dipl.Ac, LMBT, MSOM, MA
Senior Faculty, Kairos Institute of Sound Healing Goldstone Acupuncture & Whole Health

«As Dr. Christi Bonds-Garrett introduces us to the world of Vibrational Raindrop Technique, or VRT as it has been coined by her, she takes you by the hand simply and eloquently explaining each complex system that's integrated into VRT. This integration and application of principles brings healing to a powerful next level. This is an essential resource as it acquaints one with the principles to begin the journey on healing with sound, audible and inaudible. This is the starting place that will give you the tools to venture into deeper understanding of the healing process and how one may support it."

Fran Norton, RN, CCM, FCCI, CVRS

«For many years I have struggled with low back pain radiating down my legs. After receiving my first Vibrational Raindrop Technique, I was totally pain fee for 3 weeks. I could actually feel the stress/pain gently release out of my back & down my legs. What a wonderful feeling!"

Roberta Jane Clair, FCCI, BCRS, CVRS, LSH

«Dr. Bonds-Garrett, thank you, Thank You! Wow, what a difference a few days make! My back and neck had been inflamed for a month and I had tried acupuncture, chiropractic, and massage, but to no avail. After you administered the Raindrop with the tuning forks my back was a—lot better, and after a week it was completely better. That healing just creeps right up on you. That is powerful stuff! I want a set of those forks!"

Michelle Truman, Ed.D., FCCI, BCRS, LSHC

About the Author

Christi Bonds-Garrett, M.A., M.D., CAP, CCP has been offering Integrative Medical care since 1995, and has treated thousands of patients from this perspective. She received both her Master's Degree (M.A.) in Counseling and Medical Degree (M.D.) from the University of Nevada in Reno. After completing an Internship in Psychiatry in West Virginia, Dr. Bonds-Garrett completed a Residency in Family Practice in 1992, as well as becoming Board Certified in Family Medicine in 1993. For over 15 years she has specialized in Women's Health Care, utilizing unique combinations of herbs, oils, tuning forks, singing bowls and other forms of vibrational medicine to help her patients attain an optimal state of internal balance. With the publication of this book, she has completed the rigorous requirements to become a Certified Acutonics Practitioner (CAP).

While working as Medical Director for three Native American Clinics near Yosemite, California in the 1990s, she pursued advanced studies in Chinese Herbs, Nutrition, Medical Acupuncture at UCLA, and Homeopathy at the National Center of Homeopathy in Washington DC. While she lived in Nevada, Dr. Bonds-Garrett was a licensed Homeopathic Physician and testified to the Nevada State Board of Medical Examiners on behalf of the merits of Integrative Medicine.

More recently, she completed a two-year Fellowship in Integrative Medicine through the University of Arizona under the direction of Dr. Andrew Weil. While working for the Veterans Administration, Dr. Bonds-Garrett was one of a select group of twelve "Clinical Champions" nationwide for the Office of Patient Centered Care and Cultural Transformation of the Department of Veterans Affairs.

Her special interests include tapping the healing potential within through the use of creative activities. Dr. Bonds-Garrett has had multiple exhibits of her fiber art illustrating Chinese Medicine Cosmology at places ranging from colleges to city halls to art galleries. She maintains a small shop in Paducah, Heart of Healing Gallery, which specializes in textile art such as artist molas from Kuna Yala in Panama, Japanese shibori, antique Meisen kimono and elaborate uchikake (wedding kimono).